Dental Practice Health Check

Dental Practice Health Check

LESLEY BAILEY
Proprietor
Integral Business Services

Radcliffe Publishing
Oxford • New York

Radcliffe Publishing Ltd
18 Marcham Road
Abingdon
Oxon OX14 1AA
United Kingdom

www.radcliffe-oxford.com
Electronic catalogue and worldwide online ordering facility.

The use of any of the material within this book to help you manage your team and business more effectively is encouraged. However, the author or publishers cannot guarantee that the contents comply with most recent legislation and therefore advise readers that the contents are provided in an advisory capacity only and that no liability will be accepted by the author or the publishers.

British Library Cataloguing in Publication Data

A catalogue record for this book is available from the British Library.

ISBN-13: 978 1 84619 211 1

Typeset by Pindar New Zealand (Egan Reid), Auckland, New Zealand
Printed and bound by TJ International, Padstow, Cornwall, UK

Contents

Preface

The commercial world is a fluid, evolving cycle of meeting the ever-changing needs of clients. Businesses are continuously reviewing products and services and expanding their portfolios to keep pace with market trends and new developments and technology. Many dentists are adapting to the need to become more businesslike in order to maximise the potential of their practices in the same way as do any other commercial service providers.

Those businesses that are aware of these demands and are proactive in adapting their methods of service delivery to meet these needs and prepare for future ones are the ones that have the best chance of succeeding.

These days the business of dentistry is subject to the same market forces as any other business. Dentistry today is a consumer-led business where patients demand cosmetic options to help them improve the appearance of their teeth and their levels of self-confidence. If they cannot gain access to the level and scope of care and service they are seeking with you, they will go elsewhere. Some dentists find it difficult to accept that they need to provide not only dentistry that is clinically necessary, but also dentistry that the patient would like for cosmetic reasons. However, a successful dentist will provide what the patient needs and wants. It's becoming more important for dentists to recognise the requirement to offer the range of products and services to patients that are desirable, as well as clinically necessary.

Some dentists make excellent business managers, possessing the natural flair for running a profitable organisation. Many, however, lack the management skills required to enable them to lead their teams, control costs and profit margins and market their business so that it achieves its ultimate potential. This is understandable when – as is the case with so many other professions – the content of their academic course does not prepare them for running a business at all.

Experts within the profession have been heard to compare dental services with optical services in the UK and conclude that the dentistry business in the UK is 20 years behind that of its optical counterparts. I don't altogether agree with this opinion. The two businesses are very different from each other. Do you remember the name of your optometrist? Can you even remember whether you have seen the same optometrist more than once? Most of us don't remember, and more importantly, most of us don't care. The relationship we have with our dentist is altogether different. Patients will fiercely protect their relationship with their dentist. It's the number one reason why patients will sign up to a monthly payment plan – to maintain their relationship with their dentist.[1]

All professional people need something more than technical skill and experience to do their job well, but the dentist needs to develop a far greater ability in interpersonal skills to be able to truly empathise with his patient and influence the way they are feeling. The dentist needs to hone his social intelligence[2] skills and the importance of these 'soft skills' and their application is discussed at length in Chapter 7.

I think if I could sum up the definition of a good dental practice owner it would be an ethical and technically sound clinician who has acquired and developed skills in people management, business development and who has achieved all of this whilst maintaining a healthy work–life balance. Not much to ask!

And for those of you seeking this and the rewards it brings, I hope this book provides you with some of the support that you are looking for.

Lesley Bailey
August 2007

References

1 Market Research carried out and reproduced here by kind permission from Denplan Ltd.
2 Goleman D. *Social Intelligence: the new science of human relationships*. London: Hutchinson Publishing; 2006.

About the author

Lesley has more than 28 years of experience in business management, and since 1998 has worked predominantly within the dental sector.

Originally in retail management, Lesley moved into healthcare services area management with a Blue Chip organisation, before being offered a position with one of the largest and most successful dental body corporate businesses in the UK.

She went on to successfully fulfil the positions of marketing manager, operations manager, quality assurance manager and project manager and subsequently left the company in 2006 to set up her own successful company, Integral Business Services.

Lesley continues to work within dental and other business sectors, helping owners and their teams to achieve the full potential of their businesses.

About this book

I wanted to write a book that had the potential to help dental practice owners on a very practical level. In addition to sharing some sound theories and principles with you, I particularly wanted to include the practicalities of implementing them. I hope you get a tangible benefit from the book by applying some of the advice I have provided to your business model.

The content of the book will assist you in becoming a better people manager, drive your revenue and profitability through marketing and customer service and ensure your business has robust systems and procedures to support your operation. It will encourage you to step back and review your current business and establish whether, if you managed it differently, it could provide a more rewarding return for you and your colleagues. The sections on People and on Management information are particularly important to help ensure that your business functions smoothly and that you understand the key reporting areas that help you to monitor your business.

You will find that the information and advice provided will enable you to take your business to another level. There are six sections altogether:

➤ People
➤ Customers
➤ Marketing
➤ Quality management systems and procedures
➤ Management information and reporting
➤ Strategy, finance and planning.

The book is based on the areas of business I examine when completing a business health check or audits in dental and other business sectors. These key subjects represent the main areas of a business that should be functioning well in order to maximise and support revenue and profitability.

All the key aspects of running a business are covered and the content is based upon two fundamental requirements of building a profitable and successful business – the people connected with your business, be they clients or employees, and the quality of your operation to deliver your products and services consistently well.

You will find that once you have completed a health check of your business you will be able to identify the areas you need to work on and also a step-by-step pathway to achieving that change.

You can download many of the tables, audits and standard documents by logging onto www.radcliffe-oxford.com/dphc.

You can also correspond with the author by emailing info@integralbusiness services.co.uk.

Acknowledgements

I would like to thank everyone who has become involved in helping me to produce *Dental Practice Health Check*. Particular thanks to Simon Fitton from Baxter Fensham Ltd and Alan Suggett from Baker Tilly for their valued contributions. Also thank you to Clive Spring from XL Design and Marketing Consultants for his advice. Thank you to Gillian Nineham and her colleagues from Radcliffe Publishing for their support and editing skills.

People – People are your most important asset

'Coming together is a beginning, staying together is progress, and working together is success.'

HENRY FORD

Introduction

Of the seven key areas covered in this book, this one ranks as one of the most important. A good team will help you make a success of your business. It doesn't matter how robust your operation is, how strong your vision is or how well you personally care for your patients – if your team is not managed in a way that helps it to perform well as a unit and as individuals, you will find it extremely difficult to achieve your end goal.

The development of a strong team will provide a consistent level of service to your patients who like to see familiar faces at the practice each time they visit. The skills, competence and understanding your team develop whilst working together enables them to work efficiently. Loyal members of staff are good ambassadors for your business and show your patients that the practice working environment is supportive and rewarding.

It is an area that some dentists find challenging. They often don't have the time or desire to mould and develop their team. However, time invested in putting good foundations in to manage the team will be an excellent investment for the future. This chapter will show you how you can implement a number of initiatives that will help your team perform more strongly for you.

CHAPTER 1

Manage your team

Developing the framework for a good team

The dictionary defines the meaning of the word 'team' as a cooperatively functioning group of people, and 'team spirit' as an enthusiastic attitude towards working productively with a team or work group.

A team that works well together will have a positive effect upon the atmosphere within your practice and this will ultimately contribute to the profitability of your organisation. Patients relax and positively enjoy the experience of being treated by their dentist when they can see an efficient and friendly team caring for them.

The organisational structure of your team will have an impact upon how well it functions. As the principal dentist you will probably be looked upon as the team leader. Team leaders need to be consistent in their approach and are often relied on to provide strategic direction and a purpose for the business. Practice managers tend to fulfil a more tactical role, ensuring that policies and procedures are adhered to, to ensure the smooth running of the business.

Team vision

Every business should have a vision and a business plan that plots the various activities and timescales that need to be implemented to make that vision happen.

If you don't already have a vision it's a great team-building exercise to involve the team in creating the vision for your business and this could form the basis for your first extended practice meeting.

Then, once you have your business plan in place, this will keep the team focused on the vision that you have created.

You can develop your team vision by asking for statements or words that sum up what you want to achieve as a team. You may need to kick-start the session and lead the team into feeling comfortable with this process. See the example below that shows the process from the initial creative session with the team to the refinement of the team vision statement.

TEAM VISION – CREATIVE SESSION

Excellence
Quality
Successful business
Perfect smile
Harmony
Professional
Friendly
Affordable
Satisfaction

REFINED TO – TEAM VISION STATEMENT

Our team is committed to providing excellent quality care and service in a professional and friendly environment. We aim to create beautiful smiles for all our patients, both during and after treatment.

Team building

If you still feel your team lacks spirit and enthusiasm, a team-building exercise can often have the catalytic effect that generates buzz for the team, which you will need to build on using the team briefing meetings and extended meetings.

Team-building exercise

This exercise is designed to make individuals in your team think differently about their role and responsibilities within the team and about how their contribution can make a difference to staff morale, motivation and the results of the business.

➤ Arrange a team meeting, outside of normal practice hours or, if this is not possible, block half a day out of the appointment book.
➤ If possible, hold the meeting away from the practice in a neutral location.
➤ If appropriate, provide drink and snacks.
➤ Before the meeting, circulate your *Team Values Statement* (*see* Table 1.1 on p. 6) to re-establish a set of ground rules.
➤ Ask the team to think of a situation in which teamwork is important. For example, this could be:
    — Formula One racing
    — a 400-metre relay race
    — organising the Olympic Games
    — getting a new product on the shelf from design to manufacture
    — running a busy restaurant.
    — In fact, it could be anything that involves teamwork.
➤ It's more fun if you role-play this, but don't insist upon it.
➤ Spend half an hour deciding:
    — who would be required to run this team
    — what the goals of this team would be

    — what their various roles and responsibilities would be
    — what support they would require from each other
    — what might threaten their success as a team.
➤ Someone in the team should write down all the comments.
➤ At the end of this session the objective is to have a consensus of opinion on what makes a good team.
➤ Now ask the team to write down three positive things about their own team.

The next session's objective is to get the team members to *decide themselves* what they could improve in their own teamwork by adopting some of the things they identified as important in the first session.

Get the team to develop a simple action plan to take back into the practice which should form the basis for team meetings, communication. Once you have identified a way forward you must keep it going.

What's your role? Manage the process and gain the outcome you are looking for. Keep the meeting on track and try to diffuse any situations likely to damage the outcome. If you have an individual who may be disruptive, involve them in the planning of the meeting. Make them feel part of it and you may find they turn out to champion it rather than ruin it. Let the team run it and drive the outcome. You are there to facilitate it.

When teams don't function

Dysfunctional teams often report a variety of reasons why the team does not work well together, including:
➤ poor communication
➤ lack of mutual respect
➤ no recognition of effort
➤ inconsistent management style
➤ no common goal
➤ disorganisation
➤ negative or disruptive members of the team
➤ no leadership.

All teams need boundaries to define how members are expected to behave and interact with colleagues in the workplace. The team needs to set up and adopt these rules, and this exercise will be an invaluable one to help you manage your team.

The first step towards developing a strong framework for a good team is to establish your team values and ground rules. Involving the team in the development of your practice team values will create a powerful tool for you. The team is buying into the principle of agreeing to behave and respond to their colleagues in a way which is positive and mutually respectful. The values are universally applicable to everyone in the team, including the practice owner – no one is exempt. If a member of the team does not follow the team values, you have the opportunity to discuss their behaviour with them and refer them back to the team values agreed. In addition, there will be peer pressure on their colleague from other team members who have also agreed to abide by the team values.

A copy of team values must be provided to all new members of the team on day one as the minimum standard of behaviour required in your business.

TABLE 1.1 Example of team values for a dental practice team

All team members of our practice are expected to behave according to our team values. These values support the right of members to expect a supportive and constructive working environment.

> The team is responsible for defining and upholding the values set out in this document.

> The practice team leader is responsible for upholding the policy and ensuring the team members understand the importance of establishing and maintaining positive team relationships within the practice and the organisation and valuing all members of the team with equal respect.

> The practice manager is responsible for ensuring that practice teams follow the criteria set out in our team values and bases all individual and team discussions on those principles.

> All team members must take responsibility for behaving within these boundaries.

> Team values will be reviewed annually.

Team values statement

> All comments on or about the running of our dental practice will be based on observed behaviour, not on perceived attitudes.

> These comments will be based on objective evidence and how the contributor feels but will be non-judgemental.

> The focus will be on behaviours that can be changed, not wish lists.

> The aspects commented on will be those important to the effective real-time functioning of our business.

> Any questions will be genuine and not manipulative.

> All comments will be expressed from the position of self, e.g. I think . . .

> Comments should be confined only to the constructive.

> Negativity must not be allowed to flourish in the business.

> Where possible, all comments on the running of the business will be referred back to existing or previous practice behaviours by referring back to memos, minutes, etc.

> There is a need to observe everyone's personal needs and limits when offering comment or feedback on performance or contribution to the business.

> Before offering any comment or feedback, its true value to the running of the business should be clear in the participant's mind.

> All individuals within the team recognise and respect the contribution that is made to the business by all other team members.

Communication

Communication is the single most important team activity in maintaining team spirit. Be sure that, as a team, you remain committed to your overall objectives.

It is much more challenging to communicate effectively with the team in a dental business than some other businesses where there is free access to the team throughout the working day. In a dental practice, the team arrives at the practice in the morning and promptly disappears into their respective surgeries to prepare for the day. Lunchtime is often a quick dash to the shops to get back in time for the afternoon session. By the end of the day, everyone is tired and just wants to get home. So when do you communicate?

Some practices now use the messaging facility on their computer systems to communicate between work stations throughout the day. This is perfectly adequate for keeping people informed about the small day-to-day operational minutiae. It's a good idea to have an agreed protocol to ensure this facility is appropriately and professionally used, bearing in mind that patients and visitors can often openly view the messages being sent around the system. I have seen some unprofessional and inappropriate messages when visiting practices in the past!

Other practices have adopted the use of a communications book or noticeboard. This method will work provided the individual team members are made responsible for visiting the book every day or checking the noticeboards. Noticeboards do have a tendency to become a dumping area that accumulates a wide variety of information – some business related, some social and most of it out of date. If you have room and you want to have a noticeboard, consider having two. One that is kept clean, tidy and businesslike, and the other for the staff to use as they please – provided it is subject to regular housekeeping.

Practices that want to have a strong team spirit and direction should consider a daily briefing session. The briefing should be allocated 15 minutes immediately prior to the start of the morning session. The whole team must attend. As the team leader, you will run the briefing, inviting other team members to contribute where appropriate. This briefing should follow a standard pattern, providing information to the team about issues that relate directly to the business. See Table 1.2 below for a typical example of a daily team briefing. If you don't feel you can commit to a daily briefing, start with two briefings per week and review after one month to establish whether you feel it's worth increasing them to daily briefings.

The format of your daily team briefing can be tailored to meet the needs of your business. Although you could lose up to 1¼ hours of clinical time per week, which – at an average hourly rate of £200 – means it costs you £249, your business will benefit in so many ways that you will more than recover this cost. Some of the benefits include:

➤ improved team spirit means increased commitment from team
➤ there is greater focus on the product and services that drive your business
➤ you have a regular opportunity to discuss and refine operational issues to increase business efficiency

➤ there is an opportunity to acknowledge the team's efforts so the team feels recognised
➤ an educated and informed team gives them the focus in the areas that add value to your business
➤ it gives you the opportunity to reinforce your position as team leader
➤ it provides the team with opportunity to contribute positively to the business with ideas and solutions.

TABLE 1.2 Daily team briefing example

Daily team briefing
Agenda
Today's patient list: discuss any special needs that patients may have.
Review yesterday's patient list: discuss any matters arising from previous day.
Weekly running total for:
› patient sign-ups for monthly payment plan
› patient sign-ups for interest-free loans
› number and cost of 'fail to attend' and 'late cancellations'
› number of referrals (internal, external, hygiene)
› any other key performance indicator.
Compliments and patient feedback.
Issues arising.

Once a month, one hour should be blocked from the book to allow time for an extended team meeting. The extended meeting provides a slot of quality time to discuss new initiatives; review progress of the business plan (*see* Chapter 17 for business planning); inform the team of current and future marketing activity, etc.

Meetings should never be allowed to descend into grumbling sessions. A meeting I was invited to attend was not at all productive when the entire team was subjected to a tirade of moans and groans from the practice manager. The result was that the meeting became a destructive and negative experience for everyone. Issues that crop up in the day-to-day operation of the business should be dealt with as and when they occur. Meetings should leave the team feeling refreshed and reinvigorated, and re-focused on the main goals of the business.

The secret of the good performer

Have you ever stopped to wonder why some people excel within their role whilst others never quite come up to expectations?

There are three essential ingredients that we all need in order to perform well within a role or function and this section explores these ingredients and the factors that can influence them.

Focus

You understand what is expected of you, what your priorities are and the intrinsic part you play in the overall business goal.

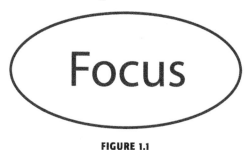

FIGURE 1.1

Any individual can only be expected to complete a task or role well if they implicitly understand what specifically is required of them and why it is required. I often come across people who are trying hard, but don't really understand what they are doing or why they are doing it.

Take the case of the dental receptionist whose task it is, every day, to telephone patients and confirm their appointment for the following day. She sees the task as a chore – a waste of time – and so often finds an excuse as to why it cannot be done, or only completes the task half-heartedly.

So is the lack of application to this task the dental receptionist's fault? After all, it's part of her job so why doesn't she just do it?

It transpires that no one has explained to the dental receptionist that the 'fail to attend' appointments are wasting over 15% of the total available time in the appointment book and that it is costing the practice more than £36k per year in lost revenue. An extra 80 patients a month could be seen during the time wasted. The additional income could be reinvested in better facilities for patients and staff.

The receptionist is set a target to reduce the percentage of 'fail to attend' appointments to less than 5% of the total time available in the appointment book. She is asked to keep track of the value of time lost from 'fail to attend' appointments and to communicate the monthly totals to patients in reception. She is also asked to implement a new policy of telephoning any patient who has failed to attend to find out why this has happened, and to issue them with a charge when appropriate.

The result is that the dental receptionist has been given the **focus** to carry out this part of her role better because she has been educated and informed and now has a target to measure her performance against. Not only does she clearly understand what task needs to be performed, but she also now understands *why* it needs to be done and why it adds value to the business and helps to meet the needs of patients.

Skill

You have the knowledge and expertise to fulfil your role and carry out necessary tasks competently.

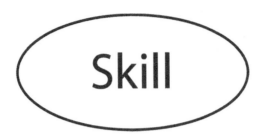

FIGURE 1.2

We are all guilty of sometimes assuming that because *we* can carry out a task or activity with ease, there should be no problem for another individual to carry out the same task with equal skill.

Skill is a combination of knowledge and experience, and having the opportunity to practise and refine a technique required to perform a task until it becomes second nature.

Imagine being given your first set of car keys at the age of 17 and being told to 'get on with it'. The chances are you will crash or stall the vehicle. The driving instructor takes his or her pupil through carefully planned stages of coaching, providing information and practical instruction until the pupil has the confidence to try what he or she has been taught, and then to practise in order to refine their driving skill until they are sufficiently competent to take their test.

The same principle applies to learning any new activity or skill. It requires someone to impart knowledge or instruction or at least to tell you where you can find information to help you. I have been to many practices where an excellent dental nurse or receptionist has been promoted into the position of practice manager without any thought being given to the new skills she will need to perform the task well.

The result is often a disaster. The new practice manager finds a whole new set of tasks she is expected to complete, but she doesn't know how to do them. She struggles to gain the authority and respect she needs to manage the team and although she completes administration tasks that keep the practice running, there is so much more she could be doing to truly drive and manage the business – if only someone would give her the skills to do it.

The combination of focus and skill together is a powerful chemistry that will help anyone perform well in their role.

Will

You have the integrity and desire to get on and do it.

The final link in the secret of the good performer is more difficult to define. How can you establish whether one of your team members is not willing to do their job well? Early warning signs can be a poor attitude, lateness, absence and disrespect for their colleagues. Can we influence a lack of will in a member of the team?

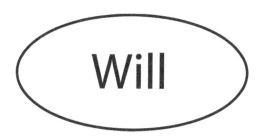

FIGURE 1.3

When I was line manager to a large team of individuals, it always worried me if a member of that team was showing a lack of will to do the job well.

As managers and leaders we have look to ourselves first and examine our own performance. If we have done our job well, all of our staff should be focused, skilled individuals. These are the first areas we should examine when we have identified a problem with someone's performance. The primary reason for an individual failing to perform well is that their manager has failed to provide them with the fundamental pieces of information and support they will require to do the job competently.

I have seen many instances of new members of staff who have plenty of will when they first start in a new role, but who unfortunately lose it through lack of training and clear direction. They become more and more disillusioned with their working environment and the satisfaction they get from going to work.

Have we provided the focus – and have we provided coaching and training to ensure they are competent to perform the tasks we have assigned to them?

If the answer is 'yes' then we must look elsewhere for the root of the problem.

The next course of action is to spend some time with the individual in a quiet area where there will be no interruptions. As caring employers we should always establish whether there are any issues going on outside of work that may be having an impact on that person's ability to perform to their usual standard. They may have become distracted because a close member of their family is ill, or they may be going through a difficult spell in a personal relationship. Whilst we all try not to bring personal problems to work, there are times when the burden placed upon an individual outside of work is so onerous that it is impossible for that person to apply themself at work, and for their spirit and ability not to be affected by the situation.

Often, just sitting, listening and empathising is enough to help that person cope better with the situation during work hours. You may agree on some holiday time or maybe a temporary reduction of hours until the situation improves. If you value that person and the contribution they have previously made to your business, you have a duty of care to them to help if you can.

If, however, there is no apparent reason for a lack of will to do the job and you are completely satisfied that you have provided them with the focus through clear instructions and the necessary training to develop their skill, the situation has to be addressed through performance management. You have established, as their line manager, that they have the focus and skill they need to do the job. You have taken time to find out whether there are any mitigating circumstances, and you realise there are not. In my experience, people who do not want to perform and who fall into this bracket are often in the wrong job or have issues with their behaviour and attitude. If these individuals are not managed appropriately, they have the capacity to infect your whole team. Other individuals will begin to resent the fact that the poor performer appears to get away with putting in the minimum amount of effort, making mistakes and being late or just not turning up. You will find it will start to affect team morale and that other members of the team may start to copy the negative behaviour (*see* Chapter 4).

It is when all three key elements of performance – focus, skill and will – are drawn together that we experience the maximum amount of value added to a business by the people working in it.

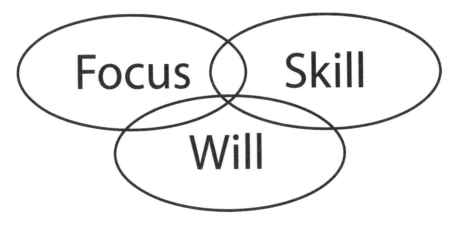

FIGURE 1.4

You will give your business a real advantage if you follow this principle with all of your team, including your associates and even yourself. You may find it useful to use the relevant sections of this book to help you develop a different approach.

Use the quick-check audit below to review how your team measures up to the 'Focus, Skill, Will' model. If you indicate any scores in column no. 1 or no. 2, you could consider developing a plan to improve your approach and enjoy the benefits that this improvement will undoubtedly bring. The list is by no means all-encompassing, but it will provide a clear indication of whether you are providing the kind of structure and culture in which your people will flourish.

TABLE 1.3 Focus, Skill, Will – quick-check audit

In the following table, column no. 1 = not at all; column no. 2 = could be better; column no. 3 = strong.

Discipline	Activity	Score		
		1	2	3
FOCUS	The team has a vision for their patients			
	The team understands and has bought into the business plan			
	All roles in the team have job descriptions			
	All roles in the team have key responsibilities			
	All roles in the team follow a standard competency model			
	All individuals have personal objectives			
	All clinicians have a personal development plan			
	The team members understand and are aware of key performance indicators			
	The team benefits from meeting targets			
	The team attends daily team briefing meetings			
	The team attends extended monthly team meetings			
	There is an annual 360° appraisal process			
SKILL	A formal staff induction programme is followed			
	An annual training and development review is completed			
	New team members are assigned a mentor			
	External resources are used to deliver regular training sessions			
	Where appropriate team members are encouraged to attend external formal training (value adding)			
	Team members are actively encouraged to share knowledge			
	There is a team succession plan			
	There are regular peer review and clinical audit sessions			
WILL	The organisation has a flat hierarchy			
	There is a democratic culture			
	Individuals are encouraged to contribute ideas			
	Constructive feedback is given to the team and individuals			
	Individuals are praised and valued for their contribution			
	There is the opportunity to progress within the organisation			
	There are clear guidelines and standards of behaviour that are consistently adhered to			
	The performance, attitude or behaviour is not allowed to flourish or go unmanaged			

cont.

Discipline	Activity	Score		
		1	2	3
WILL (cont.)	The practice has an absence policy			
	The practice has an attendance policy			
	The practice has a disciplinary process			
	The practice has a team vision			
	The practice has a team conduct policy			

It may seem like a huge task to address all of the areas listed in the table above, but this investment of your time as a leader will be good for your business. Consider the following areas in which this approach will almost certainly add value to your business:

➤ Improved cost control – team takes more responsibility for managing costs
➤ Increased revenue – better informed and more confident team sells more private options, financial plans and dental products
➤ More compliments, fewer complaints – team feels empowered to deliver consistent standards of customer service
➤ Lower staff turnover – happier team, lower stress levels, great job satisfaction
➤ Team spirit – lower stress levels, fewer mistakes improved culture.

In fact, every single aspect of your practice will be affected positively if you adopt the Focus, Skill, Will approach to managing your team.

CHAPTER 2

Recruiting staff

Starting the recruitment process

Successful recruitment is about finding the right people for your business. A few minutes' thought put into the wording of a recruitment advert or brief provided to an employment agency can save you valuable time and money. A proportion of new recruits don't stay with their new employer, many of them leaving even before their probationary period has been completed. This is often because the job does not match their expectations, or they are thrown in at the deep end and left to struggle, or a better offer has come along.

Some businesses in the dental profession suffer from a high turnover of staff. So how can you ensure you are finding the right people and – more important – retaining them? The first thing to bear in mind is the competitive state of the employment market. Some practice owners offer the basic wage with little or no additional benefits. This may save money in the short term, but can often lead to a lack of long-term commitment from your employees and you will have to bear the additional costs of having to recruit replacements each time you lose a member of your team.

Well-established teams become accustomed to working together as an efficient and cohesive unit, and it is worth paying a higher hourly rate and considering other benefits that will attract and retain quality people to your business.

Make sure the job description is accurate and indicates the level of responsibility, any flexible working hours that are required, holidays and bonuses, etc. Clearly state what experience and qualifications the successful candidate should have.

When you place the advert, be prepared to receive telephone enquiries, and make sure that you have a full job description available to send to prospective applicants. Depending upon the urgency of the appointment to fill, you may wish to dispense with some of the formalities and simply have a brief chat with applicants on the telephone before inviting them for a formal interview. You can hand out full job descriptions once you have met them, if necessary. You don't want your recruitment process to be so lengthy that it misses out on the opportunity of getting the right person simply because another practice has beaten you to it.

TABLE 2.1 Example of a recruitment advertisement for a practice manager

Practice manager

Generous salary commensurate with seniority of role

Performance-related bonus

Who are we?

We are a well-established dental practice located in a beautifully appointed, privately owned practice situated in central [Town].

We have a great team and we like to care for our patients in a positive environment.

Who are we looking for?

We are looking for an experience dental practice manager, with a proven track record in the management of a private dental business.

You are passionate in your delivery of exemplary customer service standards and are able to maximise business opportunities through effective operational, revenue and cost control.

You understand your team members and what makes them tick, so you know how to get the best from people.

What are we offering?

> excellent basic salary of 24k

> opportunity to earn additional performance-related bonus

> 25 days of paid leave annually.

The practice is open six days a week, including two late evenings.

Like to find out more?

Call in confidence on [telephone number] for an application form and job description or just to have an informal discussion, or send an e-mail to [address].

Applications to be received in writing by 30 June, to: [address].

Telephone screening

Telephone screening is an efficient way of reducing applicants and establishing a shortlist. Each prospective candidate should be asked the same questions so that you can assess each one's comparative suitability for the position. Screen all the questions you intend to ask to ensure you are complying with the requirements of age, sex and disability discrimination Acts. For example, you are no longer allowed to ask for an applicant's date of birth as doing so may be seen to be gathering information that may lead to discrimination on the grounds of age.

Questions for telephone screening

1. Tell me, what attracted you to this particular position?
2. How long have you worked in your current position?
3. What are looking to get out of the role?

4. What level of experience do you have?
5. What notice period do you have to serve?
6. Why are you looking to leave your current position?
7. What are your expectations in terms of salary?
8. What do you think you have to bring to the role that makes you the ideal candidate?

Interviews

Once the closing date for the position has passed you can review all the applications and invite candidates who have been shortlisted for interviews.

Competency and situational-based interview questions

Try to arrange to see all the candidates on the same day for interviews. If you cannot do this, try to see them over as short a period as possible. This will keep each candidate fresh in your mind. It's a good idea to have someone assisting you during the interviews. This will help you to focus on the candidates, noting body language and responses whilst your assistant makes notes of the responses given against answers from each candidate. It's also a good idea to take a photograph of each candidate as a further aide-mémoire, particularly if you have seen a large number of candidates.

It's important to put candidates at ease before commencing the formal part of the interview. This will ensure you are receiving a true reflection of the person you are interviewing.

Prepare the main questions you are going to ask before the interview and put each of these main questions to each candidate. By doing this you will get a much more balanced view when comparing their relative responses to your questions. Also note how they answer the questions and assess their body language continuously as this can reveal far more about candidates than what they are actually saying.

Competency-based questions are designed to elicit answers that provide clear evidence of competence from the candidate.

> Example
> Can you tell me about a time when you have improved a system or procedure at work?

You are looking for a specific example that illustrates what the candidate did personally. Some candidates find competency-based questions difficult and you may need to expand on the question. Give them time to consider their response and if they cannot answer it, move on to the next question.

Take into account that the candidate could be very nervous. Good candidates tend to come back to any questions they struggled with quite naturally as the interview proceeds.

Situational questions should be interspersed among the competency-based questions. A situational question is based on theory rather than a specific example.

Example

How do you manage your time effectively?

I always score the response each candidate gives to each question from 0 to 3, so that, by the end of the interviews, I can compare the responses of all the candidates and total up the score to find the overall strongest candidate.

I also spend a few minutes chatting to each candidate at the end of an interview once the formal questioning has been concluded.

You will need to give candidates the opportunity to ask questions of their own, so be prepared to know details about hours of work, holiday entitlement, other benefits, salary, start dates, uniforms, etc.

I find that the more informal part of the interview can be very revealing. For example, I once chatted informally to a prospective candidate at the end of what had been a very good interview. I asked her if she was on holiday or had taken a day off to attend the interview. She replied she had taken a day's sick leave! She didn't get the job.

Also be aware of the growing number of people who have a tendency not just to embellish their CVs, but even to fabricate them completely. I reviewed an application for a senior director's position for a SME, where the candidate with the most impressive qualifications and experience for the role had concocted a degree from an unknown university. Upon further investigation it appeared he had bought his degree online through one of the many quite legal organisations that offer this 'service'.

When you review CVs, look for gaps in employment history, or appointments taken in quick succession.

I have found that inviting the chosen candidate to spend half a day at the practice working alongside the team really works well. This is a particularly useful thing to do if you have reduced your shortlist to two candidates and cannot quite decide which one to offer the position to. It provides both parties with the opportunity to see how well you will get on together and to see how your prospective new member of staff functions in the surgery or interacts with patients. There is nothing like on-the-job observation to confirm whether or not you have made the right choice.

Managing internal promotion

A vacancy or newly created position may arise in your team that you feel can you can fill internally without the requirement to advertise externally. Care should be taken when appointing or promoting an existing member of the team to ensure team morale is not damaged as a result of poor management of the process.

The first thing to do is to let the team know that a new position is to be created within the team or that a member of the existing team is leaving. A brief job description and internal notification of application requirements for the new or vacated position and closing dates for application should be placed on the staff noticeboard and issued at the next staff briefing. Salaries and other benefits should not be made public.

TABLE 2.2 Internal recruitment advert

Practice patient co-ordinator – Opportunity

Reporting to practice manager

Internal applications are welcomed for the position of practice patient co-ordinator in the practice. Please apply in writing, enclosing a current CV and a letter to support your application, to the practice manager.

Closing date: 1 June

What does the role entail?

This is an exciting opportunity to communicate directly with patients and liaise with the clinical team to provide patients with information about treatment options.

You will be expected to discuss treatment plan financing and be able to convince patients to take up private treatment when appropriate.

You will need a good level of clinical knowledge and be able to communicate with patients using layman's language.

You will utilise practice patient literature and clinical check graphics to explain the benefits of treatment to patients.

You will have excellent customer service skills, be a good listener and be able to empathise with patients and parents of patients.

You will be self-confident and willing to work with the practice team to develop the role to its maximum potential.

Like to find out more?

Speak in confidence to the practice manager for further information.

Applications must be received in writing than no later than close of business on 1st June.

You and your practice manager need to be prepared to receive applications from members of your team whom you may not consider suitable for the post. This situation needs to be managed carefully. Should you accept their application knowing full well you have no intention of promoting them? Or should you be honest with them and turn down their application, explaining the reasons for this action? My preference is to turn down the application and explain to them that you don't feel they are quite ready for the challenge of the role. Agree on some developmental activity that will help the member of staff work towards achieving their aspirations. The easy way out is to accept the application and interview them along with everyone else, but in my experience candidates who are not ready for the role find this more demoralising than the disappointment of not being accepted for an interview. You will find your body language is very revealing to the candidate you have no intention of appointing – and what's more, they probably know that the position is too advanced for them at this stage.

Even though you may already have a clear idea of whom you will appoint, the process of advertising internally is really important as it gives everyone who is genuinely interested in the position the opportunity to express that interest. By following this process through, you will experience far less resentment in those members of the team who are not successful in their applications.

Once the appointment has been made, it needs to be formally announced to the team, together with the date when the team member will take up the new position. Sometimes people just drift into the role which causes confusion and this is not good for team spirit.

You need to make sure your newly promoted member of staff does not get carried away with his or her new responsibilities and that they are given full support in settling into their new role, particularly if it involves new line-managing responsibilities. One of the hardest things to do is to successfully achieve the move from a peer group into a position of authority and the change in team dynamics can lead to resentment if it is not sensitively managed.

Induction and probationary period
Induction

In many cases, managers tend to relax after they have successfully recruited a new staff member. The new team member is often expected to carry out all their responsibilities from day one, often with very little support. This approach sometimes works, but often results in the new recruit underperforming, making mistakes or leaving quickly.

The induction process for a new team member does not have to be very complex, but at least one day should be spent settling the new member of staff in. Ideally, this will take the form of the new recruit working alongside a colleague for part of the day, getting to know where materials and equipment are stored if they are a dental nurse, and systems and procedures if they are a receptionist/patient care co-ordinator. All new members of the team should be briefed in respect of customer service standards, team vision and the team values statement on day one. They should be familiarised with all the legal and domestic arrangements and introduced to the rest of the team at the morning team briefing.

Ensure that someone is assigned to 'buddy' up with them at lunch time so they have a companion and at the end of their first day, time should be taken to review the day and cover any questions.

TABLE 2.3 Induction – summary

Team member induction
Introductions to colleagues
Customer service standards briefed
Team member conduct briefed
Team vision briefed
Worked alongside colleague

Familiarisation of location of materials and equipment

Familiarisation of systems and procedures

Tour of the building

Emergency procedures

Commencement of shift time, breaks

Requesting time off

Reporting absence

Signing into the building

Fire regulations and appliances, fire exits, alarm

Working safely to include manual handling (bending and lifting), working with electrical appliances, responsibilities to contribute to a safe working environment

Personal security – safety at work and on the way to work

Confidentiality – patient confidentiality, practice confidentiality

Computer – maintenance of password secrecy, logging off. **Computer security rules to be read and signed with copy retained in personnel record**

Cash – accessing cash in the safe and the cash register

Training and instruction delivered by . . . .

On (date) . . . .

Areas for further instruction or improvement . . . .

Staff training record card completed . . . .

You can develop your own induction programme and go into far more depth if you wish, but sometimes it's better to have a brief introduction that you know you can deliver rather than an extended one that may be difficult to complete and becomes a burden. This brief, one-day approach helps to manage the process efficiently and also helps to manage the expectations of the new member of the team.

The induction process does not replace the ongoing training you will have to commit to, to continue to develop the new staff member's focus, skill and will – but it is a great starting point.

Probationary period

All new members of the team should be subject to a three-month probationary period. This allows you ample time to fully assess their performance, provide feedback if they need to improve in any areas, and to monitor those areas to ensure the necessary improvement has been made.

Keep a careful record of any absence during the probationary period as well as of poor timekeeping. Should any poor attendance be noted, the member of staff should be interviewed to establish the reason behind the absence or lateness.

Make sure you are providing a supportive environment in which the new member of your team can continue to learn about the role you want them to fulfil.

The line manager of the person on probation should arrange a formal monthly review of progress to date. During this meeting, both parties should be given the opportunity to discuss concerns and agree on actions and the general progress being made. If towards the end of the probationary period you remain dissatisfied with the individual's performance, you have the option of letting them go with the appropriate amount of notice, or extending the probationary period by another month and then conducting another review. If you are unsure about confirming an appointment as being permanent, then don't do so. Agree on some short-term, achievable objectives to be completed within the extended probationary period and base your final decision on your overall impression of the person's desire and ability to succeed within the role.

CHAPTER 3

Managing staff

Job titles

Referring back to page 9 in Chapter 1, bear in mind that the first key area to develop with any member of your team is *focus*.

Clarifying each job role within the team and indicating how that role contributes to the overall strategy for the business is the first step to creating a focused team.

Job titles should succinctly describe the role in question and jobs should not necessarily fall into the stereotype roles sometimes found within a practice. For example, I often recommend that the job title 'receptionist' be changed to reflect the emphasis on customer service focus. So 'Dental Receptionist' becomes 'Customer Care Co-ordinator'. Immediately the role is viewed from a different perspective – rather than the implied administrative focus of a receptionist, the customer care co-ordinator's main focus is on patients and patients also understand that the primary role of that member of your team is to look after them.

Competency definitions

Competence describes the ability of an individual to undertake the necessary activities and processes within a role to an adequate standard. You may want to consider what competencies are required across your whole business in order for it to run efficiently in every aspect. Here is a list of competencies that you may find relevant.

COMPETENCY LIST

Customer service orientation
Concern for order and quality
Clinical skill
IT and systems
Technical skills
Managing performance

Interpersonal skills
Self-confidence
Analytical skills
Business focus
Motivating and persuading

Each competency can then be broken down to a further level which illustrates specifically which criteria are applied to establish competency in each area.

Customer service orientation
➤ Develops a customer-centred business.
➤ Proactively seeks feedback from customers.
➤ Strives for constant review and enhancement of customer care standards.
➤ Ensures operational systems and procedures are contributing to positive customer experience.
➤ Leads by example and seeks daily contact with customers.
➤ Ensures colleagues represent the business in a professional manner to all third parties.

Concern for order and quality
➤ Ensures all legal and statutory requirements are complied with.
➤ Assesses and manages risk.
➤ Ensures all systems and procedures are supporting the efficient operation of the business.
➤ Ensures the core operational functions of the business are stable, using audit processes to drive continuous improvement.

Clinical skill
➤ Actively seeks to develop clinical ability.
➤ Listens to and takes on board feedback from patients and peers.
➤ Instigates and completes regular clinical self-audit.
➤ Completes required amount of CPD.
➤ Keeps up to date with new techniques and materials.
➤ Maintains a portfolio of work to chart progress and development.
➤ Investigates and takes corrective action when necessary.

IT and systems
➤ Understands the functionality of IT and systems as required to fulfil role.
➤ Ensures best practice is followed in use of IT and systems.
➤ Maintains system backups and records.
➤ Liaises with suppliers to resolve faults and install upgrades when necessary.

Technical skills

➤ Has knowledge of required techniques to operate equipment as required within role.
➤ Maintains equipment used to required standard.
➤ Maintains surgery instruments and materials to required standard.

Managing performance

➤ Ensures colleagues understand team and individual roles and aims of the business.
➤ Discusses business performance and individual contribution to the business on a daily basis.
➤ Has a formal and consistent style in reviewing performance using appraisal system.
➤ Addresses team or operational factors that have any negative impact upon the business.
➤ Has high personal standards in all aspects of the business and leads by example.

Interpersonal skills

➤ Actively listens to colleagues.
➤ Is open minded and seeks to understand underlying feelings of others.
➤ Recognises potential in colleagues.
➤ Uses intuitive skills to understand internal politics.
➤ Is compassionate and fair minded at all times.

Self-confidence

➤ Is able to deal effectively with all customers and colleagues.
➤ Is able to manage change and deal with and overcome objections.
➤ Is resilient and determined to achieve goals.
➤ Is a positive and consistent influence on team culture.
➤ Is able to address performance issues in a mature and equitable manner.
➤ Accepts criticism and welcomes feedback from customers and colleagues.
➤ Deals with and uses setbacks to achieve a positive outcome.
➤ Has high personal standards and earns respect from the team.

Analytical skills

➤ Produces business reports for self and others to track key performance indicators.
➤ Able to analyse information available from systems to conduct SWOT analysis on business and individual performance.
➤ Proactively seeks information from customers and team and executes actions based on findings.
➤ Writes and delivers reports professionally and constructively.

Business focus

- Has the desire and drive to achieve the full potential of the business.
- Has commercial awareness and understands the impact of local and global markets.
- Understands the demographics of the local market and the business and uses knowledge to drive revenue.
- Drives business expansion through internal and external marketing.
- Recognises opportunities to introduce new revenue streams and plans and implements plans to deliver them.

Motivating and persuading

- Holds regular one-to-one and group meetings.
- Ensures team individuals understand their role.
- Set challenging and realistic objectives and regularly reviews performance against those objectives.
- Uses a constructive and supportive style to deal with poor performance.
- Develops a positive team culture and spirit.
- Recognises team and individuals.
- Shares information and business goals.
- Develops skill of self and others.
- Takes on board suggestions of colleagues and recognises their contribution.
- Fosters self-belief and pride in colleagues and team.

Each role requires different competencies to be carried out capably.

Example competencies per role

DENTAL NURSE
- customer service orientation
- concern for order and quality
- technical skills
- self-confidence
- interpersonal skills.

PRACTICE MANAGER
- customer service orientation
- concern for order and quality
- IT and systems
- managing performance
- interpersonal skills
- self-confidence
- analytical skills
- business focus
- motivating and persuading.

DENTAL ASSOCIATE
➤ customer service orientation
➤ concern for order and quality
➤ IT and systems
➤ clinical skills
➤ interpersonal skills
➤ self-confidence
➤ motivating and persuading.

The competency method of building a role is a useful tool to employ when conducting training and development review, as we shall see later.

Key responsibilities

Once you have established the relevant competencies for each role within your business, the next stage is to identify the key responsibilities that accompany the role. I believe in keeping these really short and to the point so that there is complete clarity as to what is expected of the individual within that role. Don't confuse key responsibilities with the many individual tasks that have to be completed in order to fulfil the role. You may still want to provide that level of detail in the form of operational instructions that are relevant to your practice.

Example of role clarification: Dental practice manager

JOB TITLE: Dental Practice Manager
REPORTING LINE: Principal Dentist

COMPETENCIES
➤ customer service orientation
➤ concern for order and quality
➤ IT and systems
➤ managing performance
➤ interpersonal skills
➤ self-confidence
➤ analytical skills
➤ business focus
➤ motivating and persuading

KEY RESPONSIBILITIES
➤ Ensures team delivers exemplary patient care according to agreed standards.
➤ Achieves business targets through effective planning and monitoring and ensures adherence to statutory requirements.
➤ Implements, monitors and maintains standards, systems and procedures.
➤ Sets and reviews realistic goals for the business and for individuals within the business.

➤ Ensures effective teamwork and promotes morale and productivity of the team.
➤ Has a positive and optimistic approach and is able to deal with setbacks constructively.
➤ Provides quality management information for self and others, and identifies and acts upon opportunities to continuously improve performance of business.
➤ Meets revenue and profit targets.
➤ Coaches, trains and develops team individuals to help them achieve their potential.

Objective setting

If you already have your business plan in place, you can disseminate the main goals of your plan throughout the practice team by ensuring that each member of your team has a set of objectives that make a direct and tangible contribution to the goals set out in the business plan.

Objectives are also linked to the key responsibilities within each role and there should be between one and three such objectives per key responsibility. Having these will ensure that your team members continue to focus on achieving results within their role and on contributing to the overall aims of your business plan.

You will also find that if you complete this process, the burden of running the business will not rest on your shoulders alone but will be shared across the team as each objective delegates responsibility for achieving a small but important part of your business plan.

For example, here are short-term objectives for a new practice manager tasked with supporting the practice owner to address a number of areas within the business.

Example of objective setting

Objectives for Practice Manager (note those highlighted for completion with probationary period).

KEY RESPONSIBILITY 1
Ensures team delivers exemplary patient care according to agreed standards.
➤ Develop an exemplary customer experience for all patients.
➤ Monitor standards of customer service through customer focus groups and satisfaction surveys.
➤ Develop a robust complaint recovery system.
➤ Develop role of patient adviser/co-ordinator.

Objectives for three-month probation
➤ Progress the output from the patient-centred practice workshop and actively involve team in development of private patient experience by November.

➤ Develop protocols for patient co-ordinator role and involve at least two members of the team to fulfil this role by October.

KEY RESPONSIBILITY 2

Achieves business targets through effective planning and monitoring and ensures adherence to statutory requirements.

➤ Manage human resources for operational efficiency and stability.
➤ Develop and carry out a programme of internal audit to ensure best practice is delivered.
➤ Ensure operational plan is a working document to deliver key objectives in timely order.
➤ Carry out periodic risk assessment of health and safety in the practice and report findings to practice owner.
➤ Ensure good personnel practice is adhered to in all formal matters relating to employees.
➤ Ensure all necessary steps are taken to adhere to all legal requirements.

Objectives for three-month probation

➤ Present business plan to team and communicate planned developments to achieve growth and change in next financial year.
➤ Check that all critical requirements are up to date and located in core filing system by November.

KEY RESPONSIBILITY 3

Implements, monitors and maintains standards, systems and procedures.

➤ All systems to be utilised to their full functionality.
➤ Monitor all systems and procedures on ongoing basis to ensure best practice is being adhered to.
➤ Develop and maintain quality management system with colleagues to identify best practice.

Objective for three-month probation

➤ Complete an audit on signed patient consent or cross-infection control by December.

KEY RESPONSIBILITY 4

Sets and reviews realistic goals for the business and for individuals within the business.

➤ Training plan to be implemented for all colleagues.
➤ All colleagues to receive role clarification, personal objectives and annual appraisal.
➤ Business goals to be communicated at appropriate level to colleagues in monthly review meetings.

➤ One-to-one review meetings to be held with clinicians, discussing key performance indicators.

Objective for three-month probation
➤ Complete a role clarification exercise with all team members and agree objectives that relate to the business plan objectives by January.

KEY RESPONSIBILITY 5
Ensures effective teamwork and promotes morale and productivity of the team.
➤ Hold monthly practice meetings to review performance of business.
➤ Develop a staff forum to open channels of communication with colleagues, develop ideas and solve problems.
➤ Develop and maintain a communication strategy that creates a two-way, effective channel for all colleagues.
➤ Monitor and control staff costs and attendance.

Objective for three-month probation
➤ Establish your authority and management style with team by holding a team meeting in September which actively encourages team contribution and shared responsibility to achieve business development.

KEY RESPONSIBILITY 6
Has a positive and optimistic approach and is able to deal with setbacks constructively.
➤ Complete an exception report (report showing all issues arising) to track problems and outcomes, basing observations and actions on the weaknesses in processes, organisation or teamwork that caused issues arising. Produce actions to address weaknesses.
➤ Complete a self-assessment of strengths and weaknesses against competency framework and produce a personal development plan to develop areas with development needs.

Objective for three-month probation
➤ Reflect upon personal impact by maintaining a diary for one month. Consider those actions taken and responses to challenging situations and how you could have achieved a different outcome with a different style or approach.

KEY RESPONSIBILITY 7
Provides quality management information for self and others and identifies and acts upon opportunities to continuously improve performance of business.
➤ Produce a monthly key performance indicator (KPI) report showing income streams, breakdown of costs and any exceptional activity.
➤ Utilise IT software to drive hourly rates, occupancy of clinicians, take-up of treatment plans and to manage 'fail to attend' appointments and practice debt.

Objective for three-month probation:
➤ Attend a management information workshop with LB to develop ability to provide monthly KPI information to principal by November.

KEY RESPONSIBILITY 8

Meets revenue and profit targets.
➤ Working with key stakeholders, develop and deliver an operational plan.
➤ Define key targets in revenue growth and profitability.
➤ Manage all controllable costs associated with the effective running of the business to maximise profit percentage.
➤ Develop and deliver a marketing strategy to maximise potential of internal and external market place.
➤ Explore opportunities to extend existing customer offer in keeping with corporate branding and strategic direction.

Objectives for three-month probation
➤ Working with LB, devise a business plan for commencement 1 January that incorporates revenue and profit targets.
➤ Working with LB develop a marketing strategy for the first quarter of next financial year showing a breakdown of activity and approximate costs.

KEY RESPONSIBILITY 9

Coaches, trains and develops team individuals to achieve their potential.
➤ Identify key areas of responsibility for all colleagues and develop ownership of individuals.
➤ Manage unacceptable performance and behaviour in a consistent and firm manner.
➤ Undertake a skill review on an annual basis based on job competencies and key responsibilities.
➤ Develop soft skills of clinicians to maximise their ability to ethically sell to patients.
➤ Develop succession plans for all key roles.

Objective for three-month probation
➤ Meet with each clinician on a monthly basis to discuss KPI report, and other relevant issues, from January.

Although this role clarification looks a little overwhelming at first glance, in this case it provided a practice manager with a complete framework upon which to base her activities in her new role. She knew specifically what was expected of her and the timeframe for each objective. Following an initial day spent with the principal dentist clarifying her role, responsibilities and objectives, and once the principal had ensured she was comfortable with these, further support was provided through distance learning to ensure she continued to receive the assistance that she needed in order to succeed.

The practice manager's role within the practice is key to the success of the business and therefore, as the practice owner, you should be dedicating quality time with your practice manager and helping her to develop the skills she requires to drive your business. This should include regular one-to-one meetings to review the key performance indicators of your business.

Many practice managers I work with flourish and develop hugely when given the opportunity to do so. They need the focus of role clarification and objectives and the coaching and support to develop their skill. They are often the most passionate, loyal and enthusiastic workers, persevering through many difficulties.

You may find the model discussed above will help you to develop your practice manager to their full potential.

All of your team roles should have a similar model applied. Even though your dental nurses and receptionists will not have the same breadth of responsibility, they will still value and benefit from the process.

I would also encourage you to apply the same principle to your associates and dental hygienists – we will discuss this in more detail later.

CHAPTER 4

Managing staff performance

Managing poor performance

As managers we must look to ourselves if our team is failing to perform. There is a real possibility that it is the management of the team that causes the issues in performance and not the failing of the team.

Certain aspects of your own management style can help you to manage your team more effectively:

➤ respect everyone for the contribution they make to your business
➤ thank your team members and praise them for a job well done, but don't overdo it – less is more, especially when expressed sincerely
➤ don't throw money at people to appease them
➤ be consistent
➤ control your moods
➤ be a good listener
➤ admit it when you are in the wrong
➤ be firm and fair always, so your people know where they stand
➤ acknowledge the originator of good ideas and suggestions
➤ don't have favourites and don't let your head be turned by flattery
➤ always maintain a professional distance.

One of the most common comments made to me when I speak to the team in a practice is that they don't feel valued. I think this is an area that has the capacity to cause the practice owner great problems if not handled with care. Don't take on the burden of being the only person in your team who can bestow praise or value a colleague. Every team member should value the team and colleagues in the team. The most effective way of showing someone you value them is simply to look them in the eye, touch them on the arm and say, 'Thanks, well done'.

I will come back to how a management style has the capacity to influence the culture of your whole organisation in Chapter 6.

I have already discussed briefly the issues that can arise when a member of your team fails to perform to the required standard, in Chapter 1 – 'The secret of the good performer'.

Often an individual's behaviour at work will start to deteriorate if we allow it to happen. Values and standards of behaviour should be the same throughout the whole team, and the team values statement will help to cement these standards in place.

It is important to distinguish whether poor performance is due to behaviour and attitude of the individual, or to a lack of competence to carry out the tasks that are part of the role they fulfil at the practice. We have already seen the three factors – focus, skill and will – that provide the bedrock for good performance.

The first step in addressing any issue that has affected someone's performance at work is to discuss the matter with them as soon as possible. Discussions should take place away from other members of the team and should be based on establishing the facts of the matter. Voices should never be raised, and comments must be based on what has happened and not subjective personal opinions or interpretations.

Your practice manager needs to employ skills of tact and diplomacy and often a common-sense approach will resolve the matter without further action being required. It is when the situation is not addressed that resentment builds and the member of staff underperforming takes the lack of correction as an invitation to repeat the behaviour. So often a minor issue that could have been resolved with a quiet word becomes a much more unpleasant issue that is complex and time consuming to sort out. A note should be placed on the individual's personnel file to record the incident.

Your team needs to understand that standards of performance and behaviour are consistently upheld across your whole practice, so if the associate is rude to his dental nurse that is viewed with as much disapproval as when the dental nurse is rude to the associate. It is unacceptable behaviour and this should be made clear by referring the individual back to the team values statement. It should be pointed out that they are, in fact, breaking a rule they agreed to abide by. Teams respond well to boundaries and once you have established them you will find everyone appreciates the stability and consistency they provide.

If a quiet word does not have the desired effect and the situation continues, then you will need to take your action to the next and more formal level. This could involve sitting down and formally counselling the individual, or you may have to conduct a full investigation pending a disciplinary interview.

The following examples illustrate various approaches and how the issue should be escalated if the situation is not satisfactorily resolved. In all cases, notes should be taken and where necessary an assistant should be present to assist with note taking, to ensure good personnel practice is being following and to witness the content of any discussion.

Example 1

ISSUE – PERSISTENT LATENESS ARRIVING TO WORK
Process of resolution/escalation:

STAGE 1

Take member of team to one side and establish reason for lateness.

Assuming there are no mitigating circumstances, remind them of their start time and reiterate the importance of time management to ensure prompt arrival and support of colleagues.

Resolution, or . . .

STAGE 2

Continued issue with regard to timekeeping with no mitigating circumstances.

Request formal meeting to discuss unresolved issue and provide agreed timeframe to observe improvement to acceptable standard.

Inform individual that should the issue not be satisfactorily resolved in the agreed timeframe, they may be required to attend a disciplinary interview.

Resolution, or . . .

STAGE 3

Inform the individual you are holding a formal investigation as a result of their persistent lateness and failure to improve to satisfactory standard.

Complete investigation and inform person of requirement to attend disciplinary interview (*see* the disciplinary process, p. 36).

Conduct interview and consider the appropriate action.

Issue formal oral warning in writing and place copy in personnel file.

Resolution, or . . .

STAGE 4

If there is no improvement, you have no alternative but to proceed through the various stages of disciplinary process up to and including dismissal if required.

Resolution.

Example 2

ISSUE – NEW RECEPTIONIST IS MAKING A LOT OF ERRORS IN BOOKING APPOINTMENTS

STAGE 1

Hold a one-to-one meeting to establish any difficulties she may be having, and to carry out re-training.

Work alongside to ensure re-training methods have worked.

Resolution, or . . .

STAGE 2

Errors still being made.

Establish level of interest and willingness to continue in the role. Is she enjoying it? How much pressure is there to do the job – is this impacting upon her accuracy?

Complete a review of her role under her probationary period. Can she be re-assigned to other tasks to build her confidence?

Resolution, or...

STAGE 3

Errors still being made.

Complete a final review of her probationary period and decide whether to extend to give her further time to improve, or do not confirm her appointment as permanent.

Resolution.

The disciplinary process

As an employer you will know the importance of following the process of issuing disciplinary warnings to employees with extreme care. Detailed notes must be taken and retained in personnel files and each step of the process must be followed to the letter, while maintaining an objective approach at all times. The decision to issue a disciplinary warning cannot be taken until a full investigation and disciplinary interview have taken place.

Facts need to be established to see if it appears as though there is a case for investigation.

You then need to inform the individual that you are conducting an investigation. This may involve asking them or other members of the team questions and taking notes.

Once you have established the facts and have decided that a disciplinary interview should be held, you must meet with the individual involved and inform them that they are required to attend a disciplinary interview. They must have at least 24 hours' notice prior to the interview being held and must be told of their right to bring a representative with them.

The representative has no right to contribute to the interview but may make notes on behalf of the person attending the interview.

It is recommended that the interviewer also has a witness who will make detailed notes of all that is said and anything that occurs and who will ensure good personnel practice is being followed.

Once the interview commences, you must confirm that it is a disciplinary interview and what the role of each person attending it is. You must then state clearly why the interview is being held and go through the facts that you have established, listening carefully and objectively to the responses given to any questions you may have.

When you are satisfied that you have all the information you need to make an appropriate decision, you will need to suspend the interview temporarily and ask the member of staff to wait outside. This will provide you with the opportunity to fully consider your decision without being rushed.

You need to take into account a number of factors before a fair decision can be reached:

➤ is this an out-of-character incident?

➤ what bracket of misdemeanour does it fall into – minor, serious, gross misconduct (your employment contract should contain an explanation of what would
be classed as gross misconduct, but it is usually very serious breaches of
organisational policies such as drunkenness at work, proven theft, open refusal
to follow reasonable instruction, etc.).

Once you have made your decision you must call the member of staff back into the
room together with the witnesses, and summarise your findings. You must then tell
them of your decision and that this will be recorded in their file and confirmed to
them in writing.

You must also inform them they have the right to appeal against the decision
that you have made and what they need to do to make that appeal, including the
number of days (usually seven working days) they have to make an appeal. Usually
your practice manager would complete the initial stages of any disciplinary process,
in which case it would be the practice owner who would manage the appeals
process should there be one.

When this process has been completed, you should be able to continue with the
relationship and put the issue behind you, as it has been properly and completely
dealt with.

Make sure you do not use the opportunity of a disciplinary interview to raise
any other areas of the person's performance that you are not happy with. These are
separate issues and should not be included as part of this discussion.

Absence and attendance management

Some practices have ongoing problems with staff sickness. This is a costly problem
both in terms of bringing in temporary staff to cover and in terms of the increased
stress levels it causes among the remainder of the team.

If left unmanaged, it can cause serious morale issues with the rest of the team.
I advocate a strict policy of reporting absence, as follows.

➤ Absence should be reported to the practice manager directly by telephone as
soon as the member of staff knows he or she will not be able to attend work.

➤ Voicemail messages and text messages or messages left with other members of
the team are not acceptable.

➤ Upon return to work a 'return to work' interview should be conducted by the
practice manager, establishing if the individual is well enough to return and the
reason for their absence.

➤ A note will be left on their personnel file recording the relevant details of the
absence.

➤ Unacceptable levels of absence may be subject to disciplinary interview – you
are not doubting their sickness but are assessing the impact the level of absence
is having upon the business and the team.

TABLE 4.1 Absence policy

Anywhere Dental Care

Absence Policy

Anywhere Dental Care is committed to providing clear standards, policies and instructions to all its employees in respect of reporting absence from work due to illness, bereavement or other unforeseen circumstances.

All staff must follow the follow instructions when reporting an absence from work for any reason.

› Absence from work must be reported to the line manager or nominated deputy by the member of staff, in person, reporting their absence by telephone as soon as the member of staff is aware they will not be attending work.

› It is not acceptable to leave a voicemail or text message, nor to leave a message with a colleague, unless the circumstances are judged to be exceptional by the line manager.

› Upon the staff member's return to work, a 'back to work' interview will be conducted by the line manager to counsel the member of staff and establish reason for absence.

› Unacceptable levels of absence may result in disciplinary action in respect of the impact upon the rest of the team and business.

Failure to follow these instructions will result in any absence being classed as unauthorised and may result in disciplinary action being taken.

Circumstances that are judged to be exceptional by the line manager will be dealt with on an individual basis.

DP absence policy 10/06.

Similarly, tight control must be kept on annual leave for the whole team. Sometimes dentists tend to book holidays at short notice which means patients' appointments have to be cancelled.

Whilst it's reasonable to expect a dental nurse to try to get some of her holiday to coincide with that of her dentist if she has had several weeks' or months' notice, you cannot expect her to do so when only a matter of days' notice has been given.

Try to encourage a policy of holidays being spread throughout the year, and booked up as soon as possible.

Again, it's much easier to enforce rules that are already there and agreed than argue about an individual's unreasonableness.

TABLE 4.2 Annual leave policy

Anywhere Dental Practice

Annual leave policy

It is important that all members of the team have the opportunity to take their permitted annual leave. In order to ensure that the needs of the business are met whilst accommodating holiday requests, the following policy must be followed in order to gain authorisation for annual leave.

A request for booking annual leave must be placed in writing using the attached form. This form must be authorised by the line manager prior to any holidays being booked.

A copy of your authorised request will be provided to you for your records.

Annual leave entitlement should be divided evenly throughout the year; for example, one week in the spring, two in summer and one in the autumn wherever possible.

Sufficient notice period must be given to book annual leave:

> 1 week annual leave requires 1 month's notice

> 2 weeks annual leave requires 2 months' notice

> more than 2 weeks annual leave is authorised at the line manager's discretion.

You may request annual leave outside of this notice period and it may be authorised provided it accommodates the needs of the business.

Clinicians and their dental nurses should make every effort to book annual leave at the same time.

Annual leave will be authorised on a first-come-first-served basis. Verbal requests for annual leave will not be authorised unless accompanied by an annual leave request form.

TABLE 4.3 Annual leave request form

Annual leave request form

Name . . . .

Total number of days leave entitlement . . . .

From: . . . .   To: . . . .

Number of working days: . . . .

Date leave to commence: . . . .

Authorising signature: . . . .   Date: . . . .

Date leave requested: . . . .

360° review

A vital part of ensuring the ongoing development of your team is done by formally reviewing the achievement of the personal objectives they have been working on, and providing them with general feedback on their contribution to the business, while giving them the opportunity to give feedback too. Discussions should always be based on observations and fact and should remain positive and motivational. The appraisal process is not the time to tell someone they are not up to the job. Any shortfall in performance should already have been managed through ongoing performance management. Areas of concern must be discussed, but such concerns should never come as a surprise or news to the individual whose performance is being reviewed.

A lot of businesses have a robust appraisal process – on paper. When it comes to setting quality time aside to carry the process through it is sometimes a different matter in a busy practice environment. Practice managers sometimes view the process as a chore they can do without but, in fact, the process can be achieved quite quickly if the team is asked to prepare appraisal notes beforehand, together with a summary of how they have achieved their objectives. An hour should be dedicated to each member of the team, and during this time the practice manager should focus entirely on that person, meaning that telephone calls and interruptions should not be tolerated other than in an emergency. This means that if you have a staff of four, your practice manager will need to dedicate no more than a day in total to meet with each of them, review their performance and complete their training and development plan. It's quality and not quantity that counts. This investment of time will be paid back with interest as it helps to maintain the focus of your team and establishes what additional development they need to improve their skill levels and competence to do the job well.

The appraisal process also provides a non-threatening mechanism that allows people to acknowledge their weaknesses and development needs.

The first element of the process is to inform all the team members that review and training development sessions are to be completed in the forthcoming weeks. If you set a timescale, try to stick to it as it devalues the process and output if you cancel one-to-one sessions with team members.

Distribute the 360° review document (*see* example below, in Table 4.4) and allow sufficient time for team members to complete the form, together with their summary of achievements of personal objectives.

Note the positive and constructive way in which the review is structured. Don't ask people what they don't like, but instead ask them what they would like to change. You can expand the review to meet your own needs but it's often better to keep it short and to the point to manage the process efficiently.

Each member of the team should also consider which areas of their current role they need to develop and perhaps what future roles they may like to fulfil and what skills they need in order to achieve these goals. This element of the process is covered in the training and development review.

TABLE 4.4 Example of 360° review document

Name . . . .

Role . . . .

Length of service . . . .

What elements of your role do you enjoy the most?

What elements of your role would you change?

What training and development needs do you believe you have?

What elements of teamwork do you value the most?

How would you describe your feelings towards the changing needs of the business?

Summarise the results of your personal objectives and how you achieved them

Name your biggest success of this year at work

Any other comments or feedback

Competency scoring exercise

Completing a competency scoring exercise is an invaluable method of identifying the relative strengths and development needs of your team. I advocate that all members of the team – including associates and practice owners – undergo this exercise every year. Use competency definitions on pg 23–24 as you scoring template.

Each member of the team will need the list of your business competencies, together with their definitions. This will help them to position their current competence within this framework.

COMPETENCY LIST

CSO	Customer service orientation
COQ	Concern for order and quality
CS	Clinical skill
ITS	IT and systems
TS	Technical skills
MP	Managing performance
IS	Interpersonal skills
SC	Self-confidence
AS	Analytical skills
BF	Business focus
M&P	Motivating and persuading

Competency definition

Each competency can than be broken down to a further level which illustrates specifically which criteria is applied to establish competency in each area. Refer to Chapter 2 for the full breakdown of competencies.

Only the relevant competencies are selected for each role, and scores of between 0 and 3 are made against each statement that defines the competency.

➤ A score of 0 indicates no competency.
➤ A score of 1 indicates little competency.
➤ A score of 2 indicates adequate competency.
➤ A score of 3 indicates strong competency.

This exercise should be completed honestly by both the member of team and the line manager and the objective is not to point out areas in which individuals are not performing, but rather to highlight their development opportunities.

The output allows both parties to agree to a relevant and meaningful training and development programme for the following year that will add value to the business and continue to support team members in achieving their full potential.

The practice manager should ask the team to complete the exercise to provide feedback, and then the practice owner asks the practice manager to complete the exercise as well. This provides the 360° picture of your own performance and contribution to the business.

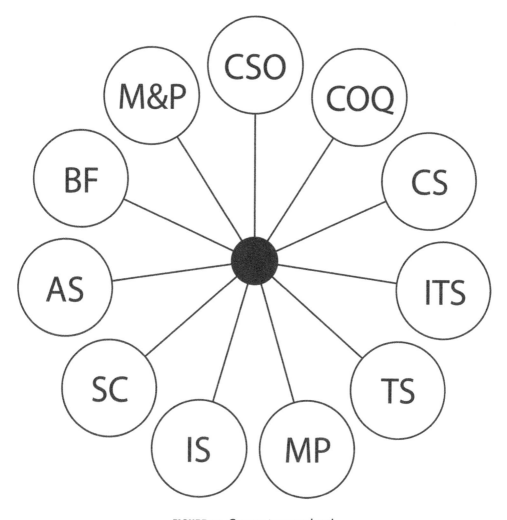

FIGURE 4.1 Competency wheel

All documents and exercises that require completion prior to the one-to-one sessions should be completed in advance and given to the reviewer to read before the meeting takes place. This maximises the value of the session, meaning the interaction is about agreeing on the results of the previous year and making plans for the forthcoming year.

By this stage of the process, the 360° review and the competency scoring exercise have been completed. You have also established what training and development each member of the team has had, and each member of your team has received formal recognition and feedback for their efforts during the previous year.

Training and development review

The formalisation of your training plan for the team and the agreeing of new objectives is a separate exercise. You will want to collate all the training needs so that you can identify common needs and arrange group training/courses accordingly. You will also want to draw up the objectives for next year from your strategic business plan. All this will be presented to the team at the appropriate time before the commencement of the next business year so as to establish new focus and renewed energy and direction.

The results of the review process may well have an impact upon team bonuses and pay reviews if you have adopted a policy of performance-related pay in your business. The final section of this chapter discusses the pros and cons of introducing incentives and bonuses to your team as well as other related team benefits.

Recognition and reward

I have previously discussed the importance of valuing the team and the contribution they make to your business. I have also touched upon the capacity for the team to manipulate you, their leader, into making greater and greater efforts to try to please them.

I have sat and listened to many miserable teams, telling me how little they feel valued and then learn that the practice owner pays generous salaries, gives Christmas bonuses, takes staff on away days and often helps out in times of personal crisis. The working conditions are good, with above-average rates of pay.

So what is the problem?

I believe one of two things may be happening in such situations.

Jealousy syndrome

I often find when I get to know the team better that there is one individual who harbours negative and bitter feelings against the practice owner. Why? Sometimes I never find out, but often it is a matter of jealousy. This member of the team started out with the practice owner and was the right-hand, trusty lieutenant. Every aspect of the business was openly discussed and plans were made and implemented. Then the business grows and the relationship inevitably changes; the practice owner develops a support network across the team and the original champion feels left out of the spotlight. The little things done that would previously have received praise go unnoticed, through no fault of the practice owner – his or her view of the business has expanded. These negative emotions are tremendously powerful and I have seen them used in very destructive ways. The practice owner is bewildered and hurt and cannot understand what has gone wrong – of course they do still value that person but in the growing family of a developing business, there's only so much attention to go round.

The fact is this individual has probably invested a great deal of commitment and effort into helping you to make the business work. Like it or not, they resent the fact that you now surround yourself with a whole network of people to continue to make it a success. Imagine it to be like a marriage: just the two of you starting out, learning lessons, working long hours to succeed. And then, because things are going so well you bring home a whole new group of people to join in – what *is* going on? You can see how personal an issue the growth of your business can become to your start-up partner. Put yourself in their position to see if you can empathise with how they are feeling.

Does this sound familiar to you? Have you seen it happen in a practice, or worse still, has it happened to you? If so, I can hear the next question forming in your mind – how can this awful situation be resolved?

When I sit down in a one-to-one meeting with a person who is in a situation like the one discussed above, they often say very similar things:

➤ 'I don't like change.'
➤ 'It's not how it used to be.'
➤ 'It used to be family and now it's all business.'
➤ 'He/she doesn't care any more.'
➤ 'I feel left behind.'

An honest two-way discussion can resolve a lot of issues. You also need to establish an appropriate role for this person so that they can retain their feelings of worth and self-esteem, whilst still adding value to your business.

For those of you who are embarking upon the challenge of becoming a practice owner, prepare your team for the evolution that will take place. Let them see your vision from day one so they feel part of it and not left by the wayside.

Different values syndrome

Ask some businessmen 'What is important to you and makes you feel good about your business?' A large proportion of them will naturally say, 'Financial reward, or the lifestyle I can enjoy from that financial reward'.

When we ask teams, 'What is important to you about your job?' Money rarely appears in the top three answers. The responses are more likely to be:

➤ recognition
➤ being valued
➤ career opportunities.

People who fall into the first category automatically assume that everyone will place financial reward at the top of their list, too. Money is an important factor to people in the second category, but they place other ideals higher. These individuals value pure financial reward less highly than they do the recognition that comes directly from their leader in the form of praise or acknowledgement of a job well done.

As human beings we naturally respond positively to attention and praise. Small gestures of encouragement and gratitude are priceless. As noted earlier in this chapter, the most effective way of showing someone you value them is simply to look them in the eye, touch them on the arm and say, 'Thanks, well done'. If you then follow that up with a financial reward that's even more positive – but crucially the personal touch is the element that adds value, and not the financial reward.

When I have challenged those teams that don't feel valued about the quality of their working environment and the generosity of their leader, their responses have been similar and somewhat shocking:

➤ 'It's peanuts to him.'
➤ 'I'd rather she just said thanks once in a while.'
➤ 'He's just bought a new car, what's £50 to him?'
➤ 'She thinks she can buy us off with cash.'

Further investigation did, in fact, show that some practice owners often forgot to say 'thank you' – and worse, sometimes treated their staff unfairly, snapping at them if they were having a bad day. So when the team grumbled about feeling undervalued, the practice owner gets a rush of guilt and remorse and does the first thing that he knows he would appreciate – financial reward.

Imagine that the goodwill you have with your team is like a bank account. You can deposit money into it and you do – every time you pay them. But you can also deposit tangible and personal acknowledgement that illustrate their value to you and the business. This will help to maintain a better equilibrium amongst the team and will enable you to draw on this 'goodwill account' again and again if you ask people to work late or cancel a day off to help out.

Again, remember not to overdo it when it comes to praise and encouragement, otherwise it becomes as meaningful as someone saying 'Have a nice day' to you in certain high-street fast-food chains.

And, most important of all, remember that recognition and valuing cuts both ways and your ultimate goal should be to create a culture in which all colleagues value and offer praise to each other, including you.

Incentives and bonuses

As the employer, you are already rewarding your team financially for doing the job you have employed them to do, so is it a good idea to introduce financial incentives, bonuses and other benefits in addition?

Bonuses can work to add further value to the business, but only if they are carefully managed. Bonuses and incentives can be very divisive and cause real friction in the team if they are not seen to reward individuals in a fair and consistent way.

Any bonus payments that are earned by the team should be shared equally across the team, pro rata to the number of hours they are contracted to work. I recommend that any bonus should reflect the difference the team has made to the business. That could be in terms of reliability and commitment, or in terms of their efforts in proactively driving the business forward. In other words, any additional payments you are making are funded entirely out of additional revenue or profit made for your business.

Reliability may take the form of a significant reduction in staff absence and therefore a considerable saving in agency fees.

Or, more positively, the contribution may be that your team has really focused on driving private treatments (with patients signing up to direct debit schemes), or introducing new products and services.

All bonuses and incentives should have formal terms and conditions to protect you and your team, so that only those that have made a contribution to the effort earn their share.

TABLE 4.5 Team bonus

Terms and conditions of team bonus
Any staff serving their notice period during the qualifying period will not qualify for bonus.
Your bonus total will be confirmed at the end of the qualifying period and you will be notified on a monthly basis of the accumulated total.
Please note that any employee with a current disciplinary record will not be entitled to receive a bonus payment.
Any bonus payments or benefits are allocated on a pro-rata basis, according to hours stated in your employment contract.
Please note that any employee on probation will not qualify for bonus until permanently appointed at the practice.
The average take-up of private treatment is based on the numbers of patients referred or self-referred to the practice and the proportion of those patients who subsequently have gone ahead with treatment. Bonus payments are awarded on take-up of private treatment over and above the practice average. The practice average will be subject to annual review.

Employee benefits

The retention of a good team means the efficiency and smooth running of your business is maintained. Every time a team member leaves and another joins, it invariably upsets the equilibrium of your business and your standards of care and service can fluctuate as a result.

Recruitment is an expensive business, whether you have advertised yourself and have invested time and effort in the interviewing and appointing process, or whether you have involved recruitment agencies who charge between 15% and 22% of the first year's salary as commission.

Turnover in the team is inevitable but if you have a good team it is worth considering what additional benefits may be offered to them as a further means to secure their loyalty to you.

Legislation gives you less flexibility to provide additional benefits for extended length of service than was previously allowed; however, there are still several options worth considering:
- pension scheme
- medical cover
- child care funding (tax efficient)
- transport and parking

➤ annual cost-of-living pay rise
➤ funding of training and further qualifications.

If you do want to use some of the principles and models illustrated in Chapters 1 and 2, remember that change is something best managed gradually over a period of time that your team is comfortable with.

CHAPTER 5

Managing your associates

Introduction

Your business has the potential to benefit enormously provided you recruit the right associate for your practice, ensuring his or her skills and experience fit in with the profile of your patients and their needs. Once you have recruited the associate, try to establish a mechanism to manage their clinical and financial performance effectively and monitor how they interact with the team and patients.

I believe there are several factors that may have a negative influence on the ability of the practice owner and practice manager to manage their dental associates:

➤ recruiting mistakes
➤ having no ground rules
➤ lack of time to give and receive feedback
➤ no time set aside for one-to-one meetings to review clinical and financial performance
➤ no communication of practice standards
➤ no defined expectations for now and the future.

All the principles discussed in Chapters 1 and 2 should be applied to your associates in exactly the same way as they are applied to your staff.

Associates have commented to me in the past, 'I am self-employed so those rules don't apply to me.' Whether your associates are employed or self-employed, it is perfectly reasonable for you to expect certain standards of behaviour and commitment to teamwork within your practice.

Recruitment

Before you consider recruiting an associate dentist, you need to consider carefully the capacity in which you are looking to take on that associate. They may be replacing an existing one and inheriting a patient list; you may be looking to pass over part of your list to them, enabling you to focus on high-end restorative and cosmetic cases, or you may be running at full capacity with the team you have and have the room and facilities to take on another associate. Are you looking for a potential partner in the long term? Are you looking for someone to develop or for someone who will be financially beneficial to your business and earn you revenue from day one? Maybe you are considering expanding the scope of treatments you currently offer and are looking to set up an associate who has specialist training and experience?

You will need to consider all of these options before you advertise the position as you will ideally only want to attract the type of associate who will be the right fit for you and your business. If you elect to use an agency for recruitment, giving them all the information will help them to select the right candidate for you – although, in my experience, some agencies will push any dentist looking for work your way and may not always follow your selection criteria.

If you do use an agency, select one with great care. Not all agencies are scrupulous organisations and I have from time to time come across situations where they will fill your vacancy and then keep in touch with the associate placed. Several months later they contact the dentist again when they may have found a better offer for them and thus 'earn' their commission all over again. Of course, the vast majority of recruitment agencies are responsible businesses. Another tip is to ensure the agency does not claim it has introduced a candidate to you when in fact it has not. This has happened to me on a number of occasions, where a dentist has telephone independently enquiring about the position he or she has seen advertised in one of the journals. They may also, coincidently, be registered with an agency. However, if the introduction does not involve the agency then it cannot claim a fee, although it may try to do so.

I have had a good deal of success advertising in the professional journals, nearly all of which now have an online vacancies section which is regularly updated.

When you start to receive applications, you can quickly shorten the list by conducting telephone interviews using the same methods previously described in recruiting your staff in Chapter 2. If you do not get the profile of dentist you are looking for, don't compromise. You are better advised to advertise again, perhaps using a different method, or to review the wording of your recruitment advert. From one month to the next, hundreds of different players enter the market for a new position. If your practice is located in an area where it is difficult to recruit, you could use some of the contacts that liaise between the UK and the European market where dentists are actively looking to move from. The Spanish, South African and German markets are particularly strong with a wide selection of clinicians, many of whom have excellent clinical and English language skills.

Before any of the candidates attend their first interview, I generally ask them to bring study models, X-rays and clinical photographs with them, together with any other examples of the standard and extent of their clinical ability and experience.

I also ask key questions that can help to establish how productive and clinically sound they are:

➤ gross hourly rate
➤ gross monthly revenue
➤ number of crowns placed per month (approximately)

➤ type of crowns placed per month
➤ types of endodontic treatment undertaken and how long they take
➤ when rubber dam is used
➤ number of referrals to specialist per month
➤ how many new patients referred to dental hygienist and what is average prescribing profile
➤ any special interests or courses completed
➤ breakdown of how they handle the patient in first consultation
➤ how long spent on patient in first consultation
➤ how long to do a crown prep
➤ prescribing profile
➤ academic interests.

Also, there are some additional questions I find useful:
➤ interests outside of work
➤ what they value in a team
➤ what contribution they have to make to teamwork
➤ how willing they are to run patient information events
➤ what their earnings need to be*
➤ notice period
➤ how they deal with complaints.

You need to tell them about:
➤ your practice standards
➤ contract percentage
➤ your expectations of an associate
➤ team ethics and culture
➤ the benefits of working in your practice
➤ the outline of the practice and profile of patients.

If your candidate shows a reaction to your practice standards and team ethics and culture that is anything other than positive, bear this in mind before you offer the position to them. Any sign of disrespect at this stage could indicate that difficulties might ensue if they join your team.

Associate contract

Once you have interviewed and offered the position, you will need to issue your new associate with a contract. It is vitally important to ensure that the contract is completely up to date in order to protect your interests.

---

* This question is very important as it will establish the rate and complexity at which your associate dentist is likely to work. If he or she only needs to earn 5k a month then they will only work hard enough to earn 5k per month.

Consider carefully the implications of all your costs before you agree percentages, since a contract negotiated with one or two percentage points in your favour will make a considerable difference to your cost of sales.

You may wish to obtain expert advice to ensure any contract issued contains all the necessary clauses.

Setting the scene

You have already explained to the successful candidate the culture and work ethic of the practice.

Now it's time to cement those principles into place. There is never a better time to establish ground rules and team standards than before you allow a new individual to become one of your team. They should feel it's a privilege to become a member of your team and should agree wholeheartedly to buy into your policies of team values, daily briefings and general commitment to respect all colleagues within the team.

You also need to establish the authority of the practice manager with the new associate. It is your practice manager who should be meeting with each associate on a monthly basis to review key performance indicators – your role as principal is to oversee their clinical performance. This is explored further in Section 5.

Prior to the contract commencing, it's a good idea to hold a meeting with the new associate and your practice manager to explain to the new associate the role of the practice manager, your role as principal dentist, and your expectations of the associate in his or her new role. This will establish lines of authority within the team and will pre-empt the associate undermining the authority of your practice manager and your position as principal dentist.

To have their agreement at this early stage will potentially safeguard you from conflict and disruption later on. Any early signs that your new team member is not abiding by your standards can be dealt with quickly.

Most importantly, should your new associate miss the first morning briefing or not contribute positively to the first monthly team meeting you must deal with the issue immediately. If you do not, you are in effect condoning his or her action and it will be more difficult to bring him or her into line in future.

Minimum standards: induction for associates

You will probably have your minimum clinical standards of care laid down in your policy documents. These might include issues such as cross-infection control, basic life support, needle stick injury, informed patient consent and the recording of contemporaneous clinical notes. Don't assume that your new associate works to the same minimum standard as you. For example, it may be your practice policy that rubber dam is used for every root canal treatment. If this is so, you need to brief your associate as some dentists do not routinely use rubber dam when carrying out this procedure.

I recommend that a small pack containing clinical standards should be prepared and provided to the new associate when his or her contract is issued. This avoids the embarrassment to you and the potential humiliation of your associate when you have to inform them on day one that their cross-infection control measures are not up to the required standard. If you have provided the information and they have chosen either to ignore it or not to abide by it, then again you have reinforced your position of authority by informing them in advance and can correct that non-adherence to standard procedure. Don't make the assumption that all qualified clinicians follow minimum standards because, unfortunately, not all of them do.

Your dental nurse is your policy administrator in the case of a new associate. She must feel that she has the opportunity to come to you or the practice manager to report any concerns she may have in terms of best practice not being followed. You can resolve any issues quickly without exposing patients, staff or your business to any risks, either through correction, or in extreme cases, dismissal. I have seen dentists not wearing gloves, taking X-rays whilst standing directly in the beam, blatantly not meeting cross-infection control standards, or placing their nurse at risk through irresponsibly discarding a used needle. So do not assume that your standards are being met until you have been reassured by the dental nurse that that is the case.

You may have also invested a great deal of time with the team developing a quality experience for patients by following a systematic method of delivering customer care. If you have a practice standard in customer service, the new associate should be briefed about this as well. Briefings should be confidently and assertively presented, making it clear that the whole practice team abides by the standards.

An important part of patient care will include the seeking of informed consent prior to the commencement of any treatment. Again, do not assume that your new associate does this as a matter of course, since many dentists do not ask patients to sign a consent form. The General Dental Council (GDC) will investigate any complaints from patients regarding lack of informed consent and whilst it may be the associate in question who is reprimanded, it will harm your reputation with your patients or within the profession if it occurs at your practice. As the practice owner, you have duty of care to ensure your associates are practising safe and ethical dentistry within statutory guidelines and minimum standards.

Make sure your new associate is aware of all the products and services that you offer, such as a monthly direct debit scheme for patients or an interest-free patient loan facility. Whilst you don't necessarily expect associates to actively sell these additional products and services, they should having a working knowledge so they can comfortably recommend them or be able to answer questions about them.

At the end of the first week, make time to hold a one-to-one meeting with your new associate. This provides the opportunity to give feedback, and for the associate, in turn, to raise any issues or queries that have arisen during that first week. If possible, the practice manager should also be present as it will be the practice manager who will continue to manage the associate from an operational point of view. Your role will be to support and manage him or her from a clinical perspective.

The most valuable and worthwhile activity you can do with your associates is to communicate with them on a regular basis. Whether that is to provide feedback and guidance or to discuss an interesting case, your proactive efforts to maintain open lines of communication with them will be extremely beneficial. They will flourish under a stewardship of clinical leadership and teamwork.

Monthly one-to-one meeting

The performance of your clinical team needs managing in just the same way as does that of your auxiliary team and your practice manager should be spending quality time with each of your associate dentists and dental hygienists to discuss the contribution they are making to patient care, team work and to the business.

If this is a completely new concept to you, you may feel slightly uncomfortable with the idea of reviewing the performance of your clinical team. It is quite reasonable to know:

a) how your revenue is being generated
b) about issues relating to teamwork and adherence to practice standards
c) how to support your clinical team to develop their skills and help them to become more successful
d) how to support your clinical team to meet the needs of their patients.

If you have a large practice, it may be too much to expect the practice manager to meet with every clinician every month. In this case, one or two members of the clinical team can be seen each month in turn.

The basis for the meeting is to provide useful and constructive feedback that will help the associate become a more effective clinician. In the case of one-to-one meetings held by your practice manager, she will be discussing in the main non-clinical issues. The clinical development of your team will be managed by you.

TABLE 5.1 One-to-one associate meeting

A typical one-to-one meeting with an associate dentist could look like this:

One-to-one meeting: associate A N Other dentist

Meeting held 23 October

Points for discussion

1. Appointments over-running – three complaints from patients last week who were kept waiting.

   Suggested solution:

   Noted by nurse that associate often commences additional work over and above that scheduled within appointment time. Suggest carry out only scheduled work and bring patient back for additional appointment. (See also Customer Service.)

2. Out of 15 new patients, only 8 referred to dental hygienist.

Suggested solution:

Remind associate of practice policy that all new patients receive hygiene referral. Will continue to monitor.

3. Hourly rate has increased from £167 to £189 in last two-month period. More restorative work now being completed.

4. Laboratory cost increased from 4% of gross revenue to 6% of gross revenue. More crown work being completed.

5. Treatment plan take-up running at 52%.

Suggested solution:

Carry out audit on patients not accepting treatment and find out why.

You will note that all points for discussion are based on fact. This enables the practice manager to broach areas of concern in an objective and constructive way. The one-to-one meetings will empower your practice manager to address issues with associates that will help to manage their performance, aid their development and increase the value they bring to your business.

Your practice manager may not yet be at the stage in her or his own development which will enable them to launch straight into this process. They may need to develop their self-confidence, analytical skills and interpersonal skills before they are ready to embark onto their first one-to-one meeting. If this is the case, allow them to conduct their first one-to-one with you as a role-play exercise.

The vast majority of associates respond extremely positively to the process, and once your practice manager has developed the new skills she may need to carry out the process, you will find your business can benefit significantly.

I also recommend that practice managers carry out one-to-one meetings with practice owners – you should also benefit from constructive and objective feedback on where you can develop you own skills.

Key performance indicators

I cover this topic in much more detail in Chapter 15 but have provided a summary here so you can see the range of topics that might be brought up in typical one-to-one sessions.

➤ Hourly rate
➤ Conversion rate
➤ Gross revenue
➤ Referral to dental hygienist
➤ Prescription to dental hygienist (clinical)
➤ Recall of patients
➤ Prescribing profile (clinical)
➤ Fail to attend and late cancellations
➤ Occupancy percentage

➤ Patient sign-up to direct debit scheme
➤ Patient sign-up to interest-free patient loan scheme
➤ Attendance of briefings and meetings
➤ Clinical audit (clinical)
➤ Continuing professional development (CPD) (clinical)
➤ Referral to specialists (clinical)
➤ Laboratory percentage to revenue
➤ Materials percentage to revenue
➤ Time keeping
➤ Complaints
➤ Clinical complaints (clinical)
➤ Compliments
➤ Teamwork

Note those areas (clinical) that would be included in any discussions you would have with your associates as clinical lead.

Your practice manager should retain a file for each associate. This will enable her, after a period of time, to identify trends of performance so that she can illustrate improvements or continued areas of concern. When you hold your monthly management meeting with your practice manager, you should allow a few minutes to discuss the one-to-one meetings so that you are fully aware and informed of any ongoing issues relating to any of your associates.

Personal development plan

We have talked about the value of creating a positive culture of performance management within the team and that your staff should all have personal objectives and a training and development plan that meets their needs.

Associates should also be encouraged to produce their own personal development plan that maps out the direction in which their career as a dentist is planned to develop and how they are going to achieve their professional aspirations. This will help you to identify what their long-terms plans are. Are they planning to continue to study to become a specialist? Do they want to maintain an academic element to their career? Are they working towards owning their own practice? Are they looking for a long-term commitment and a possible partnership?

A personal development plan for an associate is no different from a business plan for your business. It provides the opportunity for them to sit down and reflect upon the direction of their career, what they ultimately want to get out of that career and what they need to put in place to ensure they achieve it.

It will help you to plan the future of your business if you have a better idea of the direction in which your associates wish to develop. You may find a synergy in the plans you have for your business and the future aspirations of a junior associate. Or you may be able to manage the risk of losing an associate more proactively if you know well in advance what their plans are.

The content of the plan will differ depending upon what is important to each individual associate, but you may want to provide a template for them, as a guide to what they should be taking into consideration for their future development.

TABLE 5.2 Personal development plan

Example template
Area for development:. . . . .
Resource: . . . .
When: . . . .
Clinical:
Personal development:
Business:
Financial:
Personal statement:

The notion of associates providing you with their personal development plans may seem strange to start with, but in fact you are simply providing them with the direction and support they need to fulfil their personal potential in much the same way as you provide support for your team.

CHAPTER 6

Managing yourself

In the final chapter of the first section of this book, we concentrate on how you can get the best out of yourself as a business manager and leader.

Most practice owners spend very little time considering the importance of this aspect of their role. It's extremely difficult to be a key earner for the business and still find time to lead, develop and inspire your team to deliver their best for you.

Many practice owners are victims of their own success. Their practices have grown from a squat into a three- or four-surgery practice with all the strategic planning and operational requirements that are needed to keep the business developing. This is often the point when a practice owner needs support as he or she feels they have lost control of the business and the vision they had when they first started out. The ideal work–life balance can be compromised and practice owners can feel very stressed simply contemplating going into the practice, knowing the many issues that will be facing them when they get there.

Being a dental professional was much simpler when it involved turning up for work, carrying out their role as a dentist and going home again.

In order to regain that sense of being in control of your business, you may need to take yourself right back to the moment you decided you wanted to be your own boss and run your own practice. What was your vision then for the future? Do you still hold that vision today? Maybe it's changed, or maybe you just need to refocus and re-establish your vision with yourself and your team.

What is important to you?
Creating a vision

Where do you see yourself in five years' time? Sit down and examine the major aspects of your life that are positively enjoyable and ones that you want to nourish. List them, and add onto that list those new areas that you want to have the opportunity to develop.

Now complete a second list, of all those areas of your life you feel are holding you back and that you would like to be rid of or change.

Don't just limit your lists to your professional life – incorporate those areas of your life outside of work that you feel are also relevant. After all, your work and social lives are inextricably linked and so will influence each other.

Here are examples of two very different sets of lists.

Example 1

LIKE
- being own boss
- being a mother
- freedom
- being a better team leader.

WOULD LIKE TO DEVELOP
- convert practice to private
- work three days a week
- spend more time with family and friends
- enrol on implant course
- have the best reputation in town.

DON'T LIKE AND WANT TO CHANGE
- financial worries
- being stressed
- being taken out of comfort zone
- feeling as though i have lost control.

Using this example, we can see a clear vision emerging for this practice owner. By focusing on these important issues, she can start to plan both the future of her business and her personal life.

Perhaps her first objective is to enrol on the implant course as this will provide her with the opportunity to retain implant referrals at the practice. She should consider bringing in some additional help to review her financial concerns and help her address stress levels and the feeling of having lost control. She can concentrate on restorative work, perhaps bringing in another associate to take over her main list of patients. Provided the business model is acceptable, the practice can then go through a private conversion.

All of this is executed following a carefully laid out plan, in order to minimise risk and stress levels.

In this way, the practice owner achieves her short-term vision, by which time she will need to review and re-plan her original vision so she is able to move on through to the next stage in her long-term plan.

Example 2

LIKE
➤ golf
➤ holidays
➤ time with family.

WOULD LIKE TO DEVELOP
➤ more of the above.

DON'T LIKE AND WANT TO CHANGE
➤ owning my own practice
➤ managing people
➤ dentistry.

This was an extreme example; however the vision is still there. Clearly this practice owner is searching for an exit strategy that releases the goodwill from his business and provides him with the opportunity to relax and spend more time with his family.

Both these examples are equally valuable – it's what is important to *you* that matters.

What is your role?

The average human being fulfils a number of roles in their adult life. Consider for a moment all the roles that you fulfil and make a note of them, together with the amount of time you spend dedicated to each of these roles.

Example

When I completed this exercise with a client recently, nearly the whole circle was purple. This represented a significant imbalance in his work–life balance. When I suggested he should review this and try and gain a better equilibrium his response was, 'I can't, I have too much work to do'.

Steven Covey famously explored this problem in his book *Seven Best Habits of Highly Effective People*.[1] In the seventh habit, 'Sharpen Your Saw', he tells the story of a man who was walking through a wood and as he came into a clearing he noticed another man trying to saw a tree in half. The man looked exhausted. His hands were blistered and his face dripping with sweat. 'Hi, what are you doing?' asks the first man. 'What does it look like? I'm trying to saw this tree in half', replied the second man, barely looking up from the task in hand. 'Why is it taking you so long?' asks the first. 'Because I'm tired and my saw is blunt.' 'Oh! Well, why don't you have a rest and sharpen your saw?' 'Because I don't have time – I have to saw this tree in half!!'

Once you have completed this exercise it may become apparent that you need

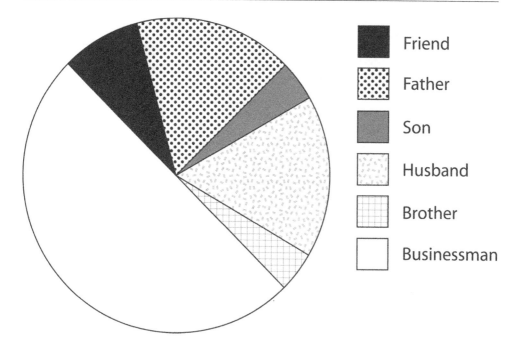

Friend

Father

Son

Husband

Brother

Businessman

FIGURE 6.1 Doughnut graph representing division of all roles as a total

some support in your business, such as a practice manager with business skills who can take the burden of the day-to-day running of the practice away from you.

Once you have established that your approach to work is healthy and you manage to fit all your other roles into your busy lifestyle, complete the same exercise; only, this time, defined by the number of roles you consider you have in your business.

Example

As potentially one of the key earners in the business, you cannot afford to spend too much time on management issues. So how do you ensure the time you do spend out of the surgery is productive and profitable for your business?

Every member of your team has a job title, competencies, key responsibilities and personal objectives to provide them with the focus and direction they need to do their job to the best of their ability. Your associates have one-to-one meetings with your practice manager, and personal development plans to keep them focused on the contribution that is expected of them in your business and on how they can work towards their ultimate potential.

As their leader, you should also have a clear idea of your role and how that role interacts with those of other members of the team. If you have committed to carrying out the daily briefings and monthly meetings, then you have already begun

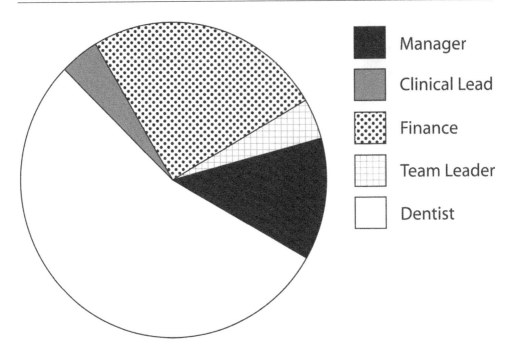

FIGURE 6.2 Doughnut graph showing division of roles within business

to illustrate to your team who their leader is. It may sound obvious – but you can only fulfil the role as leader in a visible and dynamic way.

So what exactly is your role?

Job title: Principal dentist/practice owner

COMPETENCIES
➤ customer service orientation
➤ concern for order and quality
➤ clinical skill
➤ IT and systems
➤ technical skills
➤ managing performance
➤ interpersonal skills
➤ self-confidence
➤ analytical skills
➤ business focus
➤ motivating and persuading.

KEY RESPONSIBILITIES
➤ Establish and communicate strategic direction of business.
➤ Contribute to operational and marketing plans.

> Monitor clinical standards within the practice.
> Organise and facilitate peer review and clinical audit.
> Network with local dental community.
> Conduct clinical interviews for associates and specialists.
> Establish a framework of regular formal meetings with practice manager, reviewing KPI report, operational and marketing plans.
> Share vision of business with team.
> Motivate, coach and lead the team to achieve overall business objective.
> Develop self and others to achieve personal potential.
> Manage budgets and financial performance of business.

Completion of your personal development plan, taking into account 'what is important to you' will help clarify what your role is within the organisation.

TABLE 6.1 Professional development plan

People

Instigate and hold monthly management meetings with practice manager to review financial performance of business and monitor business and marketing plan progress.

Hold monthly clinical meetings with associates to facilitate case reviews.

Foster a democratic culture within the practice, encouraging all team individuals to contribute to meetings and to the operational running of practice.

Customers

Develop ethical selling skills of self and others by attending ethical selling course.

Lead team in the development of the patient journey, taking into account your vision for the future profile of the business.

Operational

Develop more in-depth knowledge of financial performance of the business through monthly review of KPI (key performance indicator) report.

Introduce Quality Management structure to all operational processes, with regular quality process audits and required corrective action reported to you on a monthly basis by practice manager.

Marketing

Allocate annual budget for marketing plan.

Adopt and support a charity.

Review product and service development and incorporate into annual business development plan.

Develop stature and relationship with referral base.

Manage development of premises to deliver business objectives.

Strategic

Complete a review of current financial arrangements to ensure best value.

Consider options for an exit strategy and how you will get there.

Management style

If a stranger asked you to describe your management style, what would you say?

Could you describe your style as a set of ethics, values and behaviours that you have had to work hard at perfecting? Or is your style influenced by your character, your mood, your upbringing, or what has happened to you on any particular day?

Dr Daniel Goleman, whom I cite in the preface, talks about the science of human relationships in his book *Social Intelligence: the new science of human relationships*.[2] He describes two types of human interaction: nourishing and toxic. As leaders we should ensure that interactions with our teams are nourishing, and that they support the team in a consistent and positive manner.

Many practice owners describe themselves as autocratic and controlling and there is a very good reason why they have developed this style of management over a period of time. If the business has been developed from a squat, the practice owner would have been used to knowing about everything going on in the practice. As the business develops, it becomes more and more difficult to hold on to everything that is happening and eventually tasks and responsibilities are delegated to other members of the team. If this process is not managed adequately, the delegated tasks get left undone or incorrectly completed, leading to frustration for the practice owner. This often culminates in her trying to oversee everything and then feeling extremely put upon – stretched in every direction – because she cannot trust anyone to the job as well as she would have done it herself.

This situation can be resolved by re-clarifying everyone's role in the business and ensuring they have got the focus and skill to complete a task correctly. Over a period of time, the practice owner learns to trust and empower his team. It can be a liberating experience.

What group of nouns would you use to describe your character profile at work? Do others perceive you as you perceive yourself to be?

If you are not sure that the person you think you are matches the person other people think you are, try this exercise with someone you can trust to be honest.

Print off two copies of the list of the words below. Taking one list, tick against a word if you believe it does describe you and place a cross against those words that you do not think describe you. Ask your companion to carry out the same exercise using the second list. When you have completed the exercise, compare results by marking their ticks and crosses against your own.

AUTOCRATIC

MOODY

LOYAL

FUN

DRIVEN

SARCASTIC

INDISCREET

PRIVATE

INSPIRATIONAL

CHARISMATIC
UNFAIR
SENSITIVE
SERIOUS
COMPETITIVE
AMBITIOUS
RELIABLE
GENEROUS
MEAN
BAD TEMPERED
CALM
CONSISTENT
SINGLE MINDED
APPROACHABLE
HUMBLE
ARROGANT
DEMOCRATIC
EMPOWERING
CONTROLLING
MOTIVATIONAL
NEGATIVE

Now print the list off again and repeat the exercise once more, but this time place a tick against each word that you believe describes the qualities of a leader. Compare your score of ticks against your ideal.

This exercise will help you to identify areas within your behaviour that you can modify and develop to become a more effective leader of your team. No one is perfect and part of your make-up is in your character, which you should not try to change. But there are elements of your style as a manager and leader that will be affected by your behaviour, and that interaction with your team will be either nourishing or toxic.

If you reflect upon the number of toxic or negative encounters you have with your team every day, and you find that they outweigh the nourishing or positive ones, it may be time to review your management style and adapt it so that it adds value to the overall strategy of your business goal. Try to analyse what causes you stress and frustration and work through a solution.

References

1 Covey S. *The Seven Habits of Highly Effective People.* Free Press; 1989.
2 Goleman D. *Social Intelligence: the new science of human relationships.* London: Hutchinson Publishing; 2006.

SECTION 2

Customers – Your customers and the experience you give them are the future success of your business

'Your most unhappy customers are your greatest source of learning.'

BILL GATES

'To give real service you must add something which cannot be bought or measured with money, and that is sincerity and integrity.'

DONALD A ADAMS

Introduction

The expectations of customers are higher than ever and it is imperative that you understand what is important to your patients; what they value, and why they choose to come to you in preference to other providers. You also need to understand how you can improve your level of service to them. The starting point to developing your practice team to deliver truly exceptional levels of service is to first understand your patients' needs and desires and then to design a systematic method of delivering this and more each and every time they visit or contact a member of your team.

When I work with practice teams to develop their customer service, I describe 'five-star' service as being made up of dozens of layers, each representing a small act or gesture that creates value to the patient.

Every single activity that is carried out in your business should be planned and executed with the safety, comfort, convenience, and satisfaction of your patients in mind. They are central to the existence, growth and success of your business – no one is more important than the patient.

This section will help you to define what level of service is appropriate to your business and provide a framework for delivering it. We will also examine the circumstances that may mean you have to revise those standards to meet a changing need, and look at how to deal with customer service when dealing with complaint recovery.

CHAPTER 7

Establish your star rating

Where are you now?

If asked, how would your patients describe the quality of customer service they receive from you and your team? Do you know specifically what it is they value, what their likes and dislikes are? Many businesses judge the quality of service they provide by the number of written complaints they receive from their customers. If they receive no written letters of complaint in a given period of time, they assume 100% satisfaction levels. This is probably far from the true picture and the following example illustrates the importance of truly understanding the level of satisfaction of your customers.

The leading British passenger airline company British Airways commissioned a review of its customer service standards following substantial losses recorded in its financial accounts. The results of the review revealed a shocking cost to their business due to poor customer satisfaction which led the airline to fundamentally change its approach to listening to its customers and addressing complaints.

The company undertook a review of its customer service standards.

- Let us assume for this example that 1000 customers utilised the airline's services.
- Of those 1000 people, 330 (or 33%) of customers were dissatisfied.
- Of those 330, only 100 (or 23%) of customers verbally expressed their complaint.
- Of those 100, only 8 (or 8%) of customers filed a complaint to customer relations in writing.
- The group might therefore assume that 8% of customers are dissatisfied – whereas, in fact, 33% of its customers are actually dissatisfied.
- The airline thought that customer complaints cost it £47m. In fact, customer complaints cost it £423m.

The problem was the airline did not take a complaint seriously unless it found its way to the complaints department. The company did not take into account listening to and acting upon complaints at all levels within the organisation – it has subsequently empowered its teams to seek feedback from customers and deal with complaints more quickly. Now, managing complaints costs £1 per complaint to deal with but brings in £2 in additional revenue.[1]

So, firstly, you must be in a position to understand your current situation. You cannot rate your customer service standards – only your customers can do that. I ask many practice teams what their policy is on seeking feedback from patients and receiving and dealing with complaints, and I am often told, 'We don't get any'. Because we don't like to seek out criticism, we assume – unless we receive a letter of complaint or an irate telephone call – that our standards are great and nothing ever irritates our patients or affects the quality of the experience we provide them. The one or two written complaints you do get could be the tip of the iceberg, as we have seen in the example above.

Similarly, just because your patients do not complain does not mean you are delivering the kind of value-added experience that will retain their loyalty and keep them recommending your services to their friends and family. There is a huge range of difference between perfect service and poor service and it is the point within this range that you want your business to be at that will dictate just how far you will go to provide the perfect five-star experience for your patients.

If you have an incredibly busy practice that is funded by the government to provide subsidised dentistry to your patients, you need to have a realistic expectation of the lengths you can go to in this environment to deliver customer service.

Why change?

If you are intending to convert your practice to offer private treatment, your whole team will need to review the standards of customer service being delivered and establish whether these will be good enough in a private environment. Converting your business to a private practice will immediately alter your patients' expectations. Keeping people waiting or cancelling a whole afternoon session may previously have been tolerated by patients receiving treatment under the National Health Service, but you will find this will not be acceptable in private practice.

You may have decided to develop customer service standards in your practice because you are not satisfied with the current level of service you are providing, or it may be that the fundamental nature of your business is changing. If you have previously been relying on funding from the government, through subsidised dental treatment for your patients, and are now considering a conversion to independent or private practice, you will want to undertake a complete review of the quality of experience you are offering your patients.

Your business will become less intense, seeing fewer patients for longer periods of time, and your patients now paying private fees for their care and treatment will have a different level of expectation, too.

Sometimes local competition can force you to examine the quality of service you are providing and in a consumer-driven business, your patients soon disappear to the practice around the corner if they feel the quality of service there is superior. In the same way that word-of-mouth recommendations can be a great practice builder for you, they can also decimate your patient base if you are lagging behind the competition.

Before you start to develop your standards of service, complete the short benchmark audit below to help you identify the areas that may require your attention.

TABLE 7.1 Customer service audit

Tick column No. 1 if you answer 'no' to the question, if you don't know or if you are not satisfied with your current situation.

Tick column No. 2 if you can answer 'yes' to the question but are not sure you are using the information/process to its full potential or if you believe it could be improved.

Tick column No. 3 if you can answer 'yes' to the question and are confident you could not improve it in any way.

* Tick this column if you feel this area is a particular issue in your practice

Key Area 2. Customers: Your customers and the experience you give them are the future success of your business	*	✓ 1	✓ 2	✓ 3
Have you devised a 'patient journey' to ensure excellent consistent customer service?				
Do you carry out regular customer service surveys?				
Do you monitor and constantly review your product and service offering?				
Do you have a complaint recovery procedure?				
Do you spend time talking with your customers?				
Do you spend time listening to your customers?				
Do you have a method to record comments made by customers?				
Does the team receive training in customer service skills?				
Do you have a policy statement on customer service standards?				
Do you know how you compare with the competition?				
Does your approach to customer service form part of your team vision?				
Do you know how many of your new patients come from word-of-mouth referral?				
Do you know what score your customers would give you, out of five, for service?				
Do you regularly discuss your customers' experience as part of your key performance indicator report?				

If you have ticked the columns headed one and two for some of the key areas listed above, I would advise addressing each element in order of priority to help you establish good customer service standards in your business.

Gathering feedback and comments

There are various methods you can use to find out more about what your patients think of your customer service standards; what they like and dislike about coming to the dentist. Once you have gathered sufficient information about the current standards, you can use this as a basis to form a platform from which you will be able to raise standards to your preferred level.

The first, and simplest, way to gather comments from patients is to maintain a book at reception that is designed to capture any notable suggestions, comments or feedback that a patient or visitor to the practice may give. The reception team should be instructed to proactively seek comments from patients and then write those comments in the book once the patient has left. This can be done quite naturally within the scope of the normal conversation a receptionist may be having with the patient.

> **Example**
>
> 'Mrs Bailey, this was your first visit to the practice today, wasn't it? Was everything OK – how did we look after you?'
>
> 'Mr Arnold, I see you have had your crown fit done today. Are you pleased with the result?'

Any notable responses from this type of questioning should be noted in the book once the patient has left the practice and fed back to the team at daily briefings. I have seen a dental nurse glow with pride when being told in front of the whole team 'Mrs Smith says she was really nervous until Georgina held her hand and looked after her.'

Feedback requiring further investigation must be followed through without delay. You will find that this simple act of providing a mechanism for front-of-house staff to record comments adds value to the patient experience and encouragement for your team to repeat the gestures and behaviours that patients value. Already, you are becoming a more patient-centred practice. At this stage you also need to empower your team to resolve any issues raised by feedback that even just hints that the patient is dissatisfied in any way. Patients should always be thanked for the feedback they have provided as it will help you and the team to work harder to meet the needs of patients in the future.

A collation of comments over a period of time will highlight these value 'hot spots' and ensure they are repeated again and again. At the same time, issues – such as being kept waiting, not being accompanied back to reception, not being listened to – will become more important to the team members and they will try to ensure negative comments are not repeated.

In one practice where we introduced the patient comment book, it provided useful feedback on the first day. When asked if everything had been OK, the patient replied that he did not like the way the dentist spoke to his nurse. This was fed back to the dentist who now realises the embarrassment caused by disrespecting his nurse as a colleague in front of patients.

The real advantage with the patient comment book is that it can be implemented almost immediately. No special training is required and staff simply need to remember to ask patients every so often if their visit has been a positive one and whether it could have been improved upon. They can ask the questions using language they are comfortable with and in a conversational style, so they do not feel inhibited about carrying out this task. Very often individuals in the team will not comply with a change in the standards of customer service that are to be delivered because they feel uncomfortable with the actions they being asked to carry out or with the terminology they are being expected to use. Many customer service programmes originate from the United States and because of this the instructions to use certain words or phrases can make your team feel very uncomfortable. The best kind of customer service is one that is delivered sincerely and naturally.

Many coaches advocate scripting each interaction between staff and the patient. This can result in a stilted and falsely delivered quality of interface which patients find insincere. If your team is uncomfortable with the process, your patients will instinctively pick up on it and feel uncomfortable too. There is nothing wrong with asking your team to think about what they should be saying and how they could be saying it to achieve maximum impact with the patients, but I do believe in letting people express themselves in their own way, incorporating sincerity and personality into their interactions with patients. As long as the message is clear and communicated in a professional and appropriate manner that is fine, and it can develop a much stronger rapport with patients.

Satisfaction surveys

A slightly more formal approach will provide a great deal more information and this can be achieved by asking patients to complete a patient satisfaction survey. The best method to use to encourage patients to complete this is to ask them to do so whilst they are in reception. Obviously if they are a new patient they will be unable to comment except on their initial impressions (which are very important), but those patients who are attending for subsequent appointments should all be in a position to provide you with qualitative and quantitative feedback about their experience.

I do not recommend that patient satisfaction questionnaires be sent home with patients or posted out to patients' homes. You are likely to receive only a small number of completed questionnaires back. Those that you do receive back using these methods are not likely to be a fair representation of how the majority of your patients judge your customer service. There will never be a more important or relevant time for patients to provide you with feedback than when they are actually experiencing your service.

Don't make the questionnaire too long or else your patients will become bored with the process. You can tailor the questions to include information about plans for the introduction of new products and services at the practice to gauge a level of interest in these. This will prove to be useful market research that will assist you when you come to promote new services. Ensure that the reception team is fully briefed on the requirement of asking patients to complete the questionnaire. The team should know that they must explain to patients the importance of completing the questionnaire and that the findings will help the practice to meet patient needs better.

Example

You will note from the example below that one section focuses on the introduction of new products and services. Surveys can also be used to establish how patients would feel about a move to more complex restorative or specialist dentistry and, in the case of a practice receiving funding from the National Health Service (UK), how many patients would remain with the practice if it converted to private or independent practice.

TABLE 7.2 Patient survey

You are a valued patient of the practice and we like to seek your feedback and suggestions from time to time and keep you informed about new developments. This helps us to ensure that we continue to meet the needs of our patients and enables us to respond to those needs when they change.

Welcome to the Anywhere Dental Care patient survey and thank you for spending a few moments completing each question. Once you've completed the survey, please hand it in at reception.

All information provided will be classed as confidential and will not be released to third parties.

Please complete every section.

Section 1 – Patient details

Patient name

Address

Date of birth

Name of current dentist

Section 2 – Accessibility

How do you currently travel to the practice?

Walk . . . . ❏

Taxi . . . . ❏

Bus . . . . ❏

Own transport . . . . ❏

Other (please state) . . . . ❏

How would you describe parking for the practice?

Always available . . . . ❏

Not always available. . . . . ❏

cont.

Section 2 – Accessibility (*cont.*)

Are you able to gain access to the practice easily?

Yes . . . . ❑

No . . . . ❑

If you answered 'No' is this because:

The stairs are difficult for you to climb . . . . ❑

You have young children/pushchairs . . . . ❑

Are you able to make your check-up appointment easily?

Yes . . . . ❑

No . . . . ❑

Are you able to make appointments for treatment easily?

Yes . . . . ❑

No . . . . ❑

Are you able to talk to a member of the practice team when you need to by telephone?

Yes . . . . ❑

No . . . . ❑

Section 3 – Treatment

How would you describe your dental treatment at the practice?

Very good . . . . ❑

Quite good . . . . ❑

Satisfactory . . . . ❑

Not satisfactory . . . . ❑

Please provide details if you would like to:

Does the dentist see you on time?

Always . . . . ❑

Nearly always . . . . ❑

Not often . . . . ❑

Never . . . . ❑

Do we listen to your needs?

Yes, always . . . . ❑

Sometimes . . . . ❑

Never . . . . ❑

cont.

Section 3 – Treatment (*cont.*)

We are committed to providing a safe environment to treat you. How would you describe the cleanliness of the treatment rooms?

Spotless. . . . . ❏

Mostly clean . . . . ❏

Cluttered and untidy . . . . ❏

Dirty. . . . . ❏

What aspect of our service can we improve?

Section 4 – Patient plans and finance schemes

Are you aware that the practice offers the following plans to help patients spread the cost of private fees?

A. Anywhere Dental Care practice plan – a monthly direct-debit scheme to cover the cost of check-ups and which entitles patients to a reduction in private fees.

Yes, I am already a member of this plan. . . . . ❏

Yes, but I am not a member of this plan. . . . . ❏

No, I have not heard of this plan. . . . . ❏

If you are not a member of our practice plan would you like to receive more information?

Yes . . . . ❏

No . . . . ❏

B. 0% dental loan* – spread the cost of private treatment by taking out a 0% dental loan. Subject to status.

Yes, I have taken a dental loan out in the past. . . . . ❏

No, I have not heard of the dental loan plan . . . . ❏

I would like more information about a dental loan   . . . ❏

*Subject to status.

Section 5 – New products and services

We now offer an extended range of new products and services. Please indicate which of the following may be of interest to you:

Dental implants . . . . ❏

Specialist dental services . . . . ❏

In-surgery tooth whitening . . . . ❏

Invisalign – clear brace system . . . . ❏

Dental shop oral products . . . . ❏

cont.

Section 6 – Communication and development

We would like to continue to keep you informed about future plans for the practice. Please indicate which of the following are of interest:

Regular patient newsletter telling you about new developments . . . .❐

More opportunities to feed back your opinions so we can respond to the needs of
our patients more effectively . . . .❐

Access to booking appointments online . . . .❐

Confirmation of appointments using text messaging service . . . .❐

Section 7 – Any other comments

Please make any other comments that you feel will be helpful to the practice team so we can continue to meet your needs as a valued patient:

Thank you for taking time to complete this survey. Please return it to reception.

Reference

1 Horovitz J. *Service Strategy: management moves for customer results,* 2nd ed. New York: Pearson Education; 2004.

CHAPTER 8

Developing a patient-centred practice

Most teams, when asked about the level of their customer service, will give themselves a high score and it is sometimes a challenge to get them to acknowledge that this area of your business could be developed further to add value. By taking the time and trouble to draw up satisfaction surveys and asking patients to complete them, you will be able to collate the factual evidence of actual levels of patients' satisfaction After all, the score you give yourselves for customer service is irrelevant – it is the patients' perception of your service that matters.

However, you need to be aware of the implied criticism of your team by telling them that levels of customer care are not good enough. If not handled sensitively, the subject of improving customer service can often be met with comments such as:

➤ 'I can't work any harder.'
➤ 'We are already good, he's never satisfied.'
➤ 'We haven't had any complaints, so what's the problem?'

You need to emphasise the changing needs of customers and that, as a business, you want to have the very best reputation and that this means standards of customer service should be constantly under review to ensure continuous improvement. So, rather than informing your team that your customer care is poor, it can be more constructive to score this care on a scale of 1 to 10 and then aim to improve it further.

Workshop – Developing a patient-centred practice

A half-day workshop that I run is very effective in getting people in teams to think differently about the business and the role they have to play in delivering consistently excellent customer service.

There may be a local business that has exceptional levels of customer care. If your team really needs to see good customer service in action, send them out in pairs to see the best in action. Get them to discuss their findings with the rest of the team and highlight any small gestures or actions that made them feel special, or the effect visual impact upon entering a business had upon their overall impression of service.

Before you start, you will need to decide what level of customer service is realistic to aim to deliver in the profile of your practice so that you don't end up agreeing to provide a five-star experience, when it just isn't possible or realistic to do so.

Make sure that you nominate a member of the team to make notes and agree actions. The weeks that follow the workshop should be dedicated to putting into action the new customer service standards as devised and agreed by the team.

TABLE 8.1 Workshop – Developing a patient-centred practice

There is no doubt that developing the quality of patient care within the practice will create benefits for all. Not only will your patient feel tremendously valued and special, but your team will feel also good about delivering such a quality service, and your business will benefit through:

> word-of-mouth referrals

> greater acceptance of treatment plans

> increased hourly rate and profitability

> fewer complaints and more compliments

> having a team that adds true value to your business.

To begin the process of developing a patient-centred practice, the most important first step is to get the team on board and buying in to what you are committed to achieving.

Team buy-in

It's all very well to identify the standard of care and service you want to be delivered. But how can you guarantee it is delivered consistently – all day, every day – whether you are at the practice or not?

Your team have to want to do it.

To achieve this step is the most important one of all. So how?

Practice vision and team-building exercises

To focus the team on delivering the standards of care and service within your vision for a patient-centred practice, they have to understand:

> what benefits it brings to the patient

> what benefits it brings to the team

> what benefits it brings to the business and how they can enjoy a share of those benefits.

Exercise 1 – A different way of looking at service

TABLE 8.2 Exercise 1 – A different way of looking at service

This exercise is designed to remove the barriers that may hinder your team from embracing change and bringing about improvement in your service. Don't forget your team members may take your vision as an implied criticism of the standards they are already achieving, so take care to praise the level the practice is already operating at – to criticise at this stage will lead to resentment and resistance.

Get the team together – at a venue away from the practice is best, with no interruptions – but if this is not possible, block some time out and find an area of the practice suitable to gather the whole team together.

Explain the reason for the meeting – to bring the team together to create a vision for the practice and to develop a patient-centred practice. It's already noted as one of the best in the area, but we want to create the type of patient-centred practice that gives such a fantastic patient experience that no other practice will be able to compete with us.

Ice-breaker

Ask the team to list the things that are important to them when they go out for a meal to a new restaurant. You should be looking to generate a long list of things like:

> appearance of building and staff

> greeting

> toilets

> menu

> waiting staff – can they talk knowledgably about the menu; make recommendations; are they personable and friendly or haughty and cold?

> atmosphere – music, laughter, flowers

> quality of table – clean cutlery, glasses

> how the waiting staff treat you

> do you feel welcome – how, why or why not?

> service – efficient? Rushed? Kept waiting?

> food – hot, cold, presentation, appearance, flavour – served with a flourish?

> sense of theme, character, individuality of surroundings.

When you have a long list, ask the team, 'When do you start to form an impression about the quality of the food?'

Answer – as soon as you approach the building, because everything that you see or hear will be helping you to form an opinion in your mind – whether good or bad. The restaurant experience is not just about the food – it's about the whole experience.

The point is, everything single thing contributes to the experience we take away with us, and based on that experience you will return and pass on to friends the news about the great new restaurant – or do just the opposite.

The same principle applies to developing a patient-centred practice.

Every single interaction with the patient presents the opportunity to impress and contribute to the overall experience the patient goes away with.

The team should now be energetic and interactive and ready to move on to the next stage.

Exercise 2 – Why have a patient-centred practice?

TABLE 8.3 Exercise 2 – Why have a patient-centred practice?

Mini-brainstorm to establish the following:

Benefits to patients
> better informed
> feel more involved and in control
> more educated about oral health
> feel more relaxed and confident attending the practice
> feel more valued
> can make informed choices about what they want
> more funds to invest in practice comfort factor.

Benefits to team
> more motivated
> feel more valued
> more focused
> make a difference
> development of team
> receive more compliments
> feel part of a positive team culture
> share in the success of the business through team bonus scheme
> more funds to invest in equipment.

Benefits to business
> higher hourly rate
> higher acceptance of treatment plans
> higher ratio of compliments to complaints
> reputation as the best.

Exercise 3 – Creating the road map to achieve a patient-centred practice

TABLE 8.4 Exercise 3 – Creating the road map to achieve a patient-centred practice

At this stage it is worth developing some team protocols – a minimum standard that everyone commits to delivering:

> all patients to be addressed by name

> clinicians to shake hands with all patients

> appointments not cancelled by clinic except in extreme circumstances

> patients not kept waiting by clinicians

> all patient comments to be welcomed and valued

> clinician to introduce nurse to patient

> all patients will be given 100% attention by team.

You need to map the process from the first interaction the patient has with the practice to the last in any particular course of treatment.

Follow this framework:

> telephone before first visit

> first visit

> arrival at reception

> moving to consultation area

> moving to the treatment room

> return to reception

> follow-up contact.

So break down each of these milestones into its component parts, focusing all the time on opportunities to create impressions with the patient.

Decide what has to be done from an operational point of view and then layer the patient-centred approach around this. If the activity you are discussing does not benefit the patient, ask yourself why you are doing it. Does it add value to your business or is it simply a distraction?

This means concentrating on three main aspects which patients use to form their impression:

> what they see

> what they hear

> how you make them feel.

Listen to everyone's suggestions with equal interest and respect.

At this stage, you should be drawing out opportunities to promote products and services at each step of the process.

It you believe it helpful you can role-play if you wish and walk the road map as you create it.

At the end of this exercise you should have collaborated with your team and gathered ideas to develop your patient-centred practice.

This series of exercises can be completed either in one afternoon workshop or over a period of weeks, working with the team to generate enthusiasm and ideas to improve customer service and establish minimum standards that will be adopted as practice policy.

CRM – Customer Relationship Management

You have probably come across this term in other types of business-to-business scenario, but it is also a very relevant term that can be applied to the way your team manages and develops lasting relationships with your patients.

The relationship between the practice and the patient changes over time. From the initial nervous visit where certain formalities are observed to the warm and friendly, first-name greeting to 'old-timers'. I have seen this work to perfection in a practice I used to visit regularly. When I was visiting the practice a new patient arrived in great distress, having been told by a hospital that the only possible treatment for her was to have all her teeth extracted and dentures fitted. The patient was a female in her late thirties, for whom this option was a terrifying prospect. She also happened to be an extremely nervous patient, absolutely terrified of entering the surgery. She was emotional and visibly trembling with nerves, with her husband close to tears and beside himself trying to help her.

The practice manager spent time with the patient in the consultation area, with no mention of going to the surgery at all. Over a period of time she developed an understanding of her fears – mainly manifested when she felt control of her treatment was taken away from her.

I visited the practice routinely again six weeks later and was astounded to see the same patient bounce through the door as if she was going to meet a friend. There was plenty of chatter and laughter and upon seeing me the patient expressed her deep and heartfelt gratitude to the team who had invested their time wisely to develop empathy and rapport with her.

She subsequently went on to have a full mouth rehabilitation with dental implants.

That is the secret of providing good CRM to your patients. Your team knows through experience and intuition when they need to be formal and professional and when they can be more familiar. Patients perceive this change of relationship to be an indication of the value the practice team place in them.

You will find that problems that do arise with patients who have developed a 'special relationship' with your team are far easier to resolve without damage to the long-term prospects of the relationship.

You need to build into your patient-centred practice protocols, actions and gestures that help to strengthen this bond. Your patients love you to show them spontaneous gestures that illustrate how much they are valued and yet you have to plan to deliver these systematically, otherwise they may not occur naturally.

For example, when I visit my favourite restaurant with my husband or family and friends, the manager always greets us in person and shakes us by the hand. Bread and olives are delivered to our table with the manager's compliments, and at the end of the meal we are served a liqueur – again with the manager's compliments. We are always delighted as it appears we are being singled out for special treatment, but obviously this is a gesture for regular patrons that is systematically planned to have just that effect.

Think about how you and your team can identify opportunities to do the same to create added value to your patient experience.

Having a systematic approach

The next step in the process is to ensure the team has the necessary skills to deliver the standards agreed. I would also recommend that the standard of service you and your team commit to delivering during this process be incorporated into the personal objectives of all individuals so that you or your practice manager can formally review their performance against these standards during performance management and annual appraisal.

For example, if as a result of your workshop you have agreed team basic behaviours and actions that are the recognised minimum standard when greeting a patient, ensure that these are documented in a way that allows you to review an individual's performance against agreed criteria.

This translates into rules that everyone is expected to follow:

➤ positive eye contact will be made with every patient and visitor to the practice
➤ a friendly, professional smile and greeting will be given
➤ the name of the patient or visitor will be used
➤ all patients and visitors will be given 100% attention
➤ active listening techniques will be used to ensure our patients know they are being listened to
➤ associates will shake patients by the hand
➤ all team members will introduce themselves to patients and visitors by name
➤ all patients and visitors will be accompanied throughout their journey through the practice
➤ all new patients will be asked for feedback about their first visit
➤ all negative signals given out by patients will be investigated and satisfied.

These are just examples. It is important that you develop your own rules as only you and your team know the standards you can realistically deliver within the profile and intensity of your practice.

CHAPTER 9

Developing social skills

Body language and non-verbal communication

Patients and visitors to the practice will absorb a great deal of information by watching and interpreting the body language and verbal signals that we reveal subconsciously throughout our working day and our interactions with people.

It takes just four seconds to create an impression.

An amazing 93% of human communication is non-verbal. The words we say only make up a tiny proportion of effective communication:

➤ 55% of communication comes through body language
➤ 38% comes from tone, speed and inflection of voice
➤ 7% comes from what we are saying.

Our posture and facial expressions are far more revealing than we realise and can and do communicate underlying emotions and feelings to those around us.

There are several ways you can develop the awareness of your team to the power of communication through non-verbal signals.

A good starting point is to list negative body language and positive body language:

Negative body language - examples

➤ no eye contact
➤ challenging eye contact held too long
➤ impassive expression
➤ turning head away from speaker
➤ looking out of window
➤ looking at nails
➤ fiddling
➤ yawning
➤ looking at watch
➤ sniffing

- ➤ rolling eyes
- ➤ sighing
- ➤ shaking head
- ➤ shoulders slumped
- ➤ arms folded
- ➤ crossed legs
- ➤ body turned away
- ➤ closed posture
- ➤ hands clenched
- ➤ pointed finger
- ➤ eyes widening
- ➤ head down
- ➤ focus on object and not on person
- ➤ using an object as a prop to express frustration
- ➤ any repetitive physical activity – finger tapping, rubbing forehead, etc.

These are just a few of the more obvious examples that we see on a daily basis. Check out the body language signals of those around you. For example, observe at a stranger making a call on their mobile 'phone out of earshot. You will be able to tell purely from their body language whether the call is a business or a personal one. Check out a queue of people waiting to purchase lunch or a rail ticket. You will be able to tell whether they are frustrated waiting by the signals they give off.

It is really important that your team understands not only how transparent they are when they are with patients, but also how much information they can assimilate from observing your patients. If they tune into these signals it is easier to develop rapport with colleagues and clients.

Have you ever found yourself saying to a colleague, 'What's up with so-and so today?' even though that person has not spoken to you at all? Your brain has picked up in the second or two it took to pass them in the corridor that they are not in the best of moods. Your senses literally scan the facial expression, posture and response they give you like radar and judge that person's disposition based purely on that brief encounter.

This is a well-recognised human trait and patients will do just the same to you and your colleagues. So if you believe the nuances, gestures and tiny facial twitches that you use to express your feelings to your dental nurse are not also interpreted by the patient, you may be wrong. After all, they are potentially in a position which allows them the luxury of undisturbed observation.

Positive body language – examples

- ➤ smiling
- ➤ eye contact
- ➤ upright open posture
- ➤ open gestures

➤ physical contact, e.g. hand touches arm
➤ nodding
➤ head inclined towards speaker
➤ matching
➤ total focus on speaker
➤ active listening.

As human beings we are generally fascinated by the behaviour and interactions of other human beings. This is why so many people confess to enjoy 'people watching': they are interpreting the character, social standing and demeanour of strangers by piecing together observed behaviour and interactions with their companions. If you watch a young couple embrace each other in a railway station and observe their behaviour and body language as they greet each other, you will invariably find yourself smiling as you share their moment of joy. In fact, you are empathising with their mood. Your patients will behave in the same way, so a friendly and contented practice atmosphere will influence the way your patients feel and affect the overall impression they gain from their visit.

See, hear, feel

If we can sum up in three words what we should be concentrating on when developing the ideal experience for our patients they would be:
➤ what patients see
➤ what patients hear
➤ how we make them feel.

What patients see

Ask your team to take a journey around the practice, starting outside and working in pairs. Get them to write down everything that makes them feel positive about the practice environment and everything that makes them feel negative. This exercise can be greatly enhanced by inviting someone who has never been to your practice before to carry out the same activity.

They should be focusing on things such as:
➤ pavement and immediate area outside the practice should be clean of debris
➤ fascias, windows and edges of window frames clean and free of grime and maintained
➤ appearance of reception staff
➤ posters and notices up to date and professionally mounted
➤ general décor and theme, i.e. colours, pictures, displays
➤ layout of reception and seating area for patients
➤ information for patients
➤ welcoming touches such as up-to-date reading material, fresh flowers or plants
➤ general cleanliness and tidiness of reception area
➤ availability of refreshments.

As the patients proceed through to the surgery, they will continue to notice:
➤ appearance of clinical staff
➤ fresh mouthwash brought to the chairside after patient has sat down
➤ instruments unwrapped from sterile packaging in front of the patient
➤ new gloves removed from box and put on in front of patient
➤ gloves removed and discarded into bin in front of patient
➤ hands washed in front of patient
➤ dental nurse commencing cross-infection control procedures
➤ visual aids to help explain diagnosis and treatment
➤ demonstrations of oral hygiene.

You may think very few patients notice all of these indicators of excellence in your business, but many of them will notice a sufficient number to form an immediate and lasting impression about your team and your dentistry.

I went to one practice which offered quality care and service, including the placement of implants, orthodontics and tooth-whitening services. The practice owner could not understand why very few people enquired about these services. When we reviewed the outside of the building it presented a poor image of the quality of dentistry being carried out within, thus dissuading people who walked by to enter and make enquiries. The fascia was dirty and the window frames encrusted with grime from passing traffic. The pavement was littered with cigarette ends and rubbish and two small posters on the window were faded by sunlight and curling at the edges. It was not particularly noticeable to the team as they worked on the premises and had become blind to the shortfalls of the appearance of their business; however, prospective patients judged the quality of the service from the dirty façade and decided not to bother even making an enquiry.

Once you have summarised all the lists you should be able to see the areas you can emphasise to patients and those areas that require addressing and improving. Many of the negative items seen can probably be corrected quite easily and this should be done immediately. There may be other, more significant, comments such as a need for a general refurbishment of the practice that should be taken into consideration when planning capital expenditure costs in the forthcoming year.

What patients hear

Once you and the team have focused on the aspects of your business that patients see and how these may influence their impression of the quality of dentistry they may receive, you can move on to the next major area, which is what we allow patients to hear.

Your patients will expect to hear you and your team interacting with colleagues and other patients, in person and over the telephone, so what impression will they form from that experience?

Remember that 38% of human communication is made up of the tone, speed and inflection of the voice, so be mindful of these when speaking to patients or colleagues.

You can draw up another list to illustrate to the team the impression that is created for patients by what they hear.

Negative examples

➤ whispering
➤ shouting
➤ angry voices
➤ drill whirring
➤ instruments crashing together
➤ tuts and sighs
➤ exhalation
➤ other patient comments
➤ inappropriate conversations
➤ expletives
➤ telephone ringing.

Positive examples

➤ music
➤ laughter
➤ cheerful noise
➤ professional conversation
➤ people saying 'thank you'
➤ compliments from patients
➤ friendly greetings
➤ patients being addressed by name.

On the telephone

A new patient may contact your practice by telephone to make an enquiry and they will form an impression about the practice based on how the person handling their call deals with their enquiry.

The greeting should be clear and be spoken more slowly than normal conversational speed. Receptionists answer the telephone so often it is understandable that sometimes they allow the greeting to become rushed to get it out of the way. We know it takes only four seconds to create an impression, so the greeting is a vitally important component of creating a positive and welcoming impression. Ask a family member or friend to call the practice and provide you with feedback of the impression they form from an initial enquiry. They should base their observations and score on the following criteria:
➤ Was the greeting cheerful, sincere and clear?
➤ Did the person answering the telephone introduce themselves by name to the caller?
➤ Was the caller asked, 'How can I help you?'

➤ Was the caller addressed by name? That is, 'May I take your name? Thank you, Mrs Brown.'
➤ Did they feel the person answering the call had listened carefully to their enquiry and answered all questions?
➤ Was an appointment made or a contact telephone number asked for?
➤ Were they thanked for calling the practice?
➤ Was there an appropriate closing statement?

The patient waiting in reception will also overhear conversations on the telephone. Your reception team needs to be aware of this and must try to avoid conversations with suppliers or contractors at the reception desk. It will not create a positive impression if a new patient, waiting to see the dentist, has to listen to your receptionist or practice manager becoming frustrated with the engineer who was meant be at the practice repairing a faulty chair. Any conversations likely to contain any negative language or cause the receptionist to reveal frustration through body language should be made in the office.

Similarly, any patients calling with a complaint or to discuss their account should be re-routed to the office where the conversation can take place in private.

In the practice and the surgery

You will spend as much time with your colleagues as you will at home or with friends and naturally as working relationships develop in the practice, the way you speak to each other will become more familiar.

The interactions that occur between members of your team, in front of patients, should be guarded. A patient does not want to hear two receptionists discussing their romantic exploits from last weekend, nor bear witness to a dentist snapping at his nurse because something is not quite right. These incidents cause embarrassment to the patient and undermine the quality of care and service you are providing.

The patient should always be the centre of attention and never excluded from discussions relating to their care and treatment. This means the dentist should restrict the conversations he has with his dental nurse so that they relate specifically to the patient's treatment, or should involve the patient in any general conversational chat.

The most important point to remember is that, whilst the patient is lying in the dental chair, you have an ideal opportunity to educate and inform them so they can make more informed choices about the treatment options available to them.

The relationship between the dentist and the nurse in surgery should be choreographed to ensure everything the patient sees and hears reinforces the positive experience they are having.

Discussions with patients regarding financial arrangements should, wherever possible, be conducted away from the reception area. It is not appropriate to have these discussions in front of other patients. Similarly, never discuss a patient's treatment plan or dental problem in reception in front of other patients. It may be a routine conversation to you, but it's a personal and potentially sensitive issue for the patient and may prove embarrassing for other patients.

How we make the patient feel

You will develop a bond with your patients when you build rapport with them. Rapport is developed by being attuned to each person's individual need. We begin the process of developing rapport when we understand how our body language and non-verbal communication influence the feelings and emotional state of others.

As a team focused on delivering excellent customer service to your patients, your first priority is to make each patient feel valued and special as an individual.

In addition to employing the techniques we have already discussed, you can further enhance the opportunity to develop rapport by being aware of the body language the patient is exhibiting and what that is revealing about the way they are feeling.

Matching

Matching is the term that describes putting someone at ease by mirroring their body language. We all do it to some extent naturally and some of us are better at it than others – usually those people who seem to develop rapport rapidly are naturally good at this technique. For others it takes practice and a concerted effort.

When you escort your patient to the consultation room/treatment room for the first time, show them to a comfortable chair and sit opposite them. The chairs should be at the same level and so you are not too close to each other (we all have 1.5 m of personal space we are sensitive to). You will immediately be able to see the benefit of matching the seated posture of the patient rather than towering over them whilst they lie supine in the dental chair. They will be put at ease and feel more comfortable telling you what is important to them about their dental care.

If the patient's stance is open and expansive then your stance should be the same – if they are the opposite, you should adjust your stance to put them at their ease.

We all use this technique when we talk to a small child, by squatting down to match their height and reduce the possibility of intimidating them.

Pacing

We often confuse each other and misunderstandings can occur when we use different words to communicate.

Pacing means we repeat key words and phrases back to the patient, using exactly the same language as they do. This sends a subconscious message to the patient that you have heard and understood what they have said.

It's particularly useful to identify needs and deal effectively with complaints.

Example
Patient: 'So how much is the home tooth-whitening kit?'

Dentist: 'We take impressions first and then the bleaching agent and trays are £350.'

Patient: 'Right . . . but how much is the home tooth-whitening kit?'

Or

Patient: 'So how much is the home tooth-whitening kit?'

Dentist: 'The home tooth-whitening kit is £350, and that includes everything you will need.'

Patient: 'That sounds good to me . . .'

WITYA

This is a great tool to help you quickly understand what your patients want.

Ask, 'What is important to you about . . .?'

If you ask this question, you will maximise the benefit of time spent at the consultation appointment. Some dentists try to give far too much information to the patient and they leave the practice bewildered and confused, never to return.

When you meet your new patient for the first time, establish their desires quickly by asking this question.

It is also a useful question to ask to bring closure to a complaint.

That is, ask, 'So what is important to you so we can resolve your complaint?'

Overcoming objections

Sometimes it is useful to provide the team members with techniques to help them to manage potentially challenging situations.

Feel, Felt, Found

> **Example**
> Patient: 'I think it's very expensive to have private dental care.'
>
> Dentist: 'I understand how you **feel** about the cost of the private dental care. Some of my other patients have told me they have **felt** like that too, but when I explain that I can spend more time on my patient's dental needs, use better materials and dental laboratories and generally offer a much superior service, they **found** that private dental fees are actually excellent value.'

This technique works well because you are developing empathy with the patient. You are telling him or her that it is fine to feel this way and that they are not isolated in these feelings because other patients have felt that way too. Finally, you are dealing effectively with their objections by illustrating that the other people who also expressed those feelings were reassured when things were properly explained to them.

CHAPTER 10

Recovery planning

Complaint management

Patients who complain are friends, not enemies, and provided you and your team have a proactive approach to not just manage complaints when they occur but also to seek them out, your team will be able to deal confidently and successfully with 99% of all complaints.

We know through market research that people who complain are actually indicating they want to remain with you as a customer and are providing you with the opportunity to correct the mistake that has occurred. Thirty-seven per cent of people who do voice a complaint come back, whereas only 9% of people who are unhappy with the service they have received but do not complain come back.

Complaints should be seen as 'free' information provided by patients to help you improve the quality of your service and, for this reason, the member of your team dealing with the complaint should thank the patient for bringing the issue to your attention.

One of the biggest causes of complaints getting out of hand is that there is often no sense of ownership or empowerment among members of your team to deal effectively with the problem. This can lead to the patient being passed on to another member of the team when they are asked to repeat their complaint about the problem all over again. This results in a growing sense of frustration for the patient and a complaint that may have been relatively minor and that could have been dealt with by the first member of the team being told about it, develops into an ongoing issue that – as far as the patient is concerned – no one wants to deal with.

The first course of action is to establish a culture in your business whereby all your team members are encouraged to proactively seek feedback from patients. When that feedback involves even the smallest negative comment, the member of staff dealing with that patient should:

➤ Thank the patient for bringing it to your attention. 'Dr Brown will be very grateful that you have pointed that out to us. Thank you for taking the trouble to do so, Ms Green.'

➤ Establish what action, if any, is required to satisfy the complaint. 'What is important to you so you feel we have addressed your complaint?'

You will often find that just listening to your patients' complaints with 100% attention and thanking them for bringing these matters to your attention will fully satisfy the patient that you have taken their complaint seriously and that you intend to act upon it.

It is important to recognise when your patient reaches the point where they feel the wrong has been corrected, and your team must pursue any complaint with this objective in mind.

Some complaints may seem petty and rather unimportant when you and your team are trying to run a busy dental practice, but don't underestimate the power of dealing with a complaint effectively. If you handle the situation well, many complaints are opportunities to win patients for life.

So that your team feel empowered to deal with complaints, you will need to establish what level of authority individuals need to resolve the complaint, and what they need to do if the situation exceeds that authority level.

It is possible to pre-empt a complaint by tuning into the non-verbal signals being communicated by a patient. For example, a patient glancing at the clock and appearing restless may well be indicating he or she is getting impatient waiting for their appointment. Rather than ignore this behaviour, the receptionist could go and sit next to the patient and explain that 'Dr Booth is running a little late, caring for another patient. I am sorry to keep you waiting, will this cause you a problem today?'

The majority of people will appreciate the calm and honest approach, whilst those who truly cannot be kept waiting at least have the opportunity to arrange another appointment before they have reached the point where they have had to express their dissatisfaction. Circumstances like these, which can occur on a regular basis, also provide an opportunity to offer excellent customer service.

'If you have any shopping to do or errands to run, I could call you or send you a text message to let you know when to return to the practice if that is helpful.'

Many patients would be delighted by this thoughtful gesture and the situation has been reversed into a positive experience for the patient.

It is important to show patients you genuinely care about their problem. This can be achieved by building rapport with them as shown earlier in this chapter. Once you have listened carefully to the problem and taken notes, if required, you may not be able to resolve the issue immediately. In cases like this you need to inform the complainant what you intend to do and when you intend to do it, together with confirmation of when you will let them know the outcome of your investigation.

Then ensure that you follow through on all of your commitments to resolve the complaint.

Different types of people complain in different ways and it is useful to know these types and how they behave and how to deal with them effectively. To identify each type, observe their behaviour and actively listen to them with 100% of your attention. Find out what is important to them to achieve resolution and ensure notes are taken. By following the whole process through, 99% of complaints can be resolved in a positive and constructive way.

Quality controller

Between 20% and 30% of people who complain fit into this behaviour type. They like to tell you where you are going wrong and will probably tell you about a time when they excelled in this particular area.

When you have completed the investigation, write to the patient explaining how you have improved your systems and procedures and thanking them for taking the time to raise the matter with you.

Negotiator

Between 20% and 25% of complaints will come from negotiators. They are looking for something to compensate them for the experience they have received. Find out what they would value to compensate them for their trouble and thank them for raising the matter with you, but do not allow them to bargain.

Victim

Victims want empathy and you can expect 15% to 20% of people who complain to fall into this type. Develop empathy with them using the 'feel, felt, found' technique explained in Chapter 9 – 'I can understand how you feel, I would have felt that way too . . .' Thank them for raising the issue.

Reasoner

The reasoner is a logical person who wants an explanation as to what has gone wrong, and why it has gone wrong. About 20% to 25% of complaints will come from reasoners. Explain what system you have in place and why, on this occasion, it has gone wrong. Also say what you are doing to prevent the same problem re-occurring. Thank them for raising the issue.

Fan

Between 5% and 20% of complaints will come from fans. These individuals are seeking approval and recognition for identifying the issue. Emphasise how grateful you are that they have raised the issue and that they are the first person to bring it to your attention.

The unreasonable complainant

Even when complaints are handled to the best of your team's ability, you will occasionally come across aggressive and abusive patients who don't know how to express their issues in a reasonable way.

People who behave in this manner within your business need to be dealt with firmly and calmly, given one chance to modify their behaviour and then de-registered from your practice if they do not.

If your practice is in an area where you seem to have to tolerate a lot of rude and aggressive patients, display your policy on aggression for all to see.

TABLE 10.1 Policy on aggression

Policy on aggression

The staff and associates working at this practice have the right to work in a safe environment.

We are committed to treating our patients and colleagues with courtesy and respect at all times.

We expect our patients to treat us as they would wish to be treated.

Patients behaving in an aggressive or threatening manner will be de-registered from the practice with immediate effect and will be requested to leave the premises.

Make it clear to your team members what they should and should not tolerate. This will help them deal much more confidently with an unpleasant situation should it occur.

No one should be made to accept verbal or physically threatening behaviour as part of their job in a dental practice.

Patients who do start becoming abusive should be shown the policy on aggression. Confirm to them that, whilst their complaint is important, it will only be addressed when their behaviour is modified and deemed acceptable.

On no account allow any member of your team to become isolated in a situation of this nature. Remain calm and professional at all times.

Marketing – Maximise the opportunity to promote your business

---

*'In marketing I've seen only one strategy that can't miss
– and that is to market to your best customers first, your
best prospects second and the rest of the world last.'*

JOHN ROMERO

CHAPTER 11

Internal marketing

Introduction

Every business needs to promote its products and services through marketing. This aspect of growing your business is becoming more important as your competitors may use every opportunity to communicate and promote their brand and services to prospective patients and it's easy to get left behind by the new spas and cosmetic surgeries and their smart new images.

There are many different methods of marketing that can be used to bring new patients into your practice and this section will look at some of these ideas and how to plan your marketing strategy, prepare to market, and measure your success. You will also note that marketing your business need not necessarily be a costly exercise. Many internal marketing opportunities involve little or no investment except in training the team to recognise and act upon business opportunities.

Maximising internal marketing opportunities

The most powerful and cost-effective form of marketing is carried out within the practice. It is vital to ensure that your teams are well trained in the art of positive communication and ethical selling. Many practices find their best referral source is word-of-mouth recommendations from existing patients. This makes the experience you provide patients a vitally important marketing tool and the quality of service and care delivered will enable you to grow your business organically without the need for expensive marketing.

Communication

Whilst you may not necessarily want your team to overtly sell your products and services, you will want them to listen to and understand the needs of patients so they can make the most appropriate recommendations to them and provide them with relevant information.

Information displayed in windows or throughout the practice should be professional, up to date and well maintained. If you are lucky enough to have a window, you can promote your business very effectively to passing traffic. Even a first-floor surgery can attract new patients with clear signage. Make sure your window communicates the quality of your service and the type of treatments you carry out at the practice. Promote the areas of dentistry that patients shop around for, such as tooth whitening or other cosmetic treatments. Ensure your brand, products and services are clearly communicated – don't assume that just because *you* know it's a dental practice, passing traffic will also know this.

Case study

I provided support and marketing advice to a large private practice situated in one of the biggest cities in the UK. The practice was beautifully appointed, and near to the city centre with excellent passing pedestrian and vehicular traffic. It was a green-field site that had been opened for over three years and was yet to make a profit for the practice owner because of the lack of new patients registering at the practice – on average between 10 and 15 each month. This number is not sufficient to support a private practice where the numbers of new patients registering needs to be between 30 and 40 per month in order to grow the business.

The practice had a large window that filled almost the entire frontage of the premises, which were located at street level. It was part of a large office block that had shops and offices on the ground floor. To understand why the numbers of new patients were so small, I first checked the new patient referral report which showed the highest proportion of new patients were in fact passing by the practice, mainly on foot. We then conducted a street survey, stopping passers-by and enquiring whether they knew what type of business was being run from the premises. Out of 50 passers-by asked the question, an amazing 43 said they did not know or were not sure what business was run from the premises.

The practice owner had elected to furbish the business to an extremely high standard and used a contemporary, minimalist style to create a sophisticated and beautiful setting for dentistry. It was this decision that appeared to confuse the passers-by. I commissioned a full-colour, full-size design that covered the window completely. Included within the design was lettering describing the practice and the range of dentistry carried out there. A cut-out in the design allowed for a poster to be displayed in the window, meaning new promotions could be changed regularly to provide an area for interesting and new information.

Following the installation, the number of new patients who registered at the practice increased to over 30 per month. Within the first week of the new window design being completed, three new patients who worked in the office block immediately above the premises registered, and commented how convenient it was that there was a new dentist near to their place of work.

Communication mechanisms

Every piece of printed or e-mailed material that reaches your patients or third parties should be designed and written to support and strengthen your brand. Take time to print everything off your computer system, gather all your leaflets together and compare the quality, style and layout of text. Even the font size and style should remain standard.

Many practices now use a questionnaire when the patient registers at the practice to gather important information about the patient's desires and concerns relating to their dental health. Your clinical team can then use this information as the basis of the initial conversation held during the first, critically important consultation.

Example questionnaire

YOUR INITIAL CONSULTATION

We are pleased to welcome you to Anywhere Dental Care. At your first consultation you will be seen by a fully qualified and experienced dentist, who will advise and treat your specific condition and will take care to ensure you are comfortable and cared for during your consultation.

When you arrive at the practice, you will be welcomed by one of our care team who will confirm your details are entered correctly on our computerised practice system and ensure you are comfortably seated in our reception area that has a range of reading material and relaxing music. Cloakrooms are provided for your comfort and convenience.

The dentist will want to establish what is important to you about your dental care prior to completing your oral assessment and diagnosis, including the taking of any necessary diagnostic radiographs, and then he or she will discuss all possible treatment options with you, to ensure you can make informed choices about your dental treatment.

Our team of carers and clinicians continually strive to provide the very best service to our patients and are committed to providing you with a range of treatment options to enable you to make an informed choice about your dental treatment. In order to assist us in this task, it would be most helpful if you would consider and respond to the following questions and then bring them with you to your consultation. This will help us to establish what is important to you with regard to your dental treatment.

What is important to you about your treatment?
Are you currently experiencing discomfort due to your oral condition?
Yes   ☐
No   ☐

Are you able to eat, talk and laugh with confidence?
Yes   ☐
No   ☐

Are your teeth sensitive to heat_____ cold_____ ?

Do your gums bleed when you brush your teeth?
Yes ☐
No ☐

Do you have any anxiety about attending the dentist?
Yes ☐
No ☐

Please add any other factors which are important to you, or any other information that will enable us to care for you as an individual

. . . .
. . . .
. . . .
. . . .
. . . .

There is an opportunity to provide a wide variety of information to patients whilst they are waiting to be collected from reception. This information may take the form of the practice brochure, a portfolio of 'before' and 'after' photos, or an educational DVD. Your reception team should also be encouraged to interact with new patients, making them feel welcome and helping them to complete their medical history form if they have not already done so. Some practices even have a portfolio of all the 'thank you' cards they have received to illustrate how many satisfied and happy patients they have treated in the past. If you elect to do this, it's advisable to seek permission from the patients sending cards before placing the cards on open display.

Visual aids are a good tool to use to illustrate your explanation to a patient during their examination. If you do not have access to an intra-oral camera, a mirror can be used to show your patient particular areas of concern. Some dentists who do have intra-oral cameras do not use them regularly. If you do have access to one, use it for every new patient to help you communicate more effectively.

Once you have completed the initial examination and taken any necessary radiographs, you will need to present your treatment plan to the patient in a confident manner, clearly illustrating the options for treatment and the benefits they will bring. If you do not enjoy discussing the financial arrangements needed to proceed with treatment, you could consider appointing a patient co-ordinator to carry out this task.

Some dentists find it difficult to 'close the deal' with patients and in situations like this it may help to develop a framework to follow for all new patients. This will help to ensure you tell the patient the information they need to hear and to ensure you do not confuse them with too much information at their first visit.

Example: Framework for first consultation

➤ introduction
➤ what is important to you?
➤ examination with detailed commentary
➤ explanation and treatment plan
➤ financial arrangements
➤ next appointment.

One of the most important areas to consider is that it is not wise to judge the patient's ability to pay for private treatment by their appearance, age or apparent social standing.

Ensure your practice team is well informed and comfortable with the general promotion of products and services to patients in the practice and enquiries they receive over the telephone. For example, if you have a good display and stock of oral hygiene products, your dental hygienist should be actively recommending those products that will be beneficial to your patients. A private practice with three surgeries can easily generate 12 to 15k of sales in this area annually.

The contact details of all telephone enquiries should be taken and recorded and relevant information posted to the enquirer. The call should be followed up a week later as a courtesy to ensure they received the information and to answer any further queries. If your front of house team lack confidence in 'selling' or feel at all inhibited about promoting your professional services this will certainly damage your business and the numbers of new patients registering with you.

I conduct 'mystery shopping' surveys for clients when there is a significant difference between the numbers of enquiries compared to the number of new patient consultations.

Case study

A practice that needed to increase the numbers of new registrations asked for my assistance. The first task was to introduce a simple procedure that required the team to record the number of telephone enquiries, the reason for each person's call, and whether they made an appointment. On average, between 25 and 30 enquiries were taken from callers each month, but the number going on to book an appointment was always less than half this number. This figure was disappointingly low and I needed to understand what was preventing callers, who were clearly interested in what the practice had to offer, from making an appointment.

The results revealed the problem to be a lack of product knowledge, confidence and desire on the part of the front-of-house team to promote the business. When my 'mystery shopper' called to make enquiries about tooth whitening, the first time she was told, 'Before we go any further, I need to tell you this is a private practice.' The receptionist then listed the costs of the initial consultation and hygiene appointment. She could not explain what the tooth-whitening treatment would entail. My caller had been instructed to ask about interest-free payment plans that would help spread the cost of the treatment. She was asked to call back the following day when the practice manager would be able to help her. When she called back the next day, she was told there was no such plan at the practice – information which was, in fact, incorrect.

This is an extreme example; however, it does illustrate that the power of internal marketing lies in the ability of your team to communicate with patients. The team members must know what products and services are available and must be able to talk to patients in layman's terms about the treatment they may expect to receive. They also need to overcome any reticence they have in working within a private practice to ensure any negative feelings they may have are not communicated to patients.

Investing in external marketing in a business where staff are poorly trained and the experience provided to patients is not well planned and delivered is potentially a complete waste of money. Ensure you have maximised the internal marketing opportunities before you invest in any external activity so you have the confidence that the new patients you do attract to the practice will receive exceptional care and service. This will mean that they, in turn, will promote your business through word-of-mouth referral.

Patient co-ordinator role

The development of one or more of your team to fulfil the role of patient co-ordinator can significantly add value to your business. The patient co-ordinator can spend quality time with the patient, answering any questions that may have arisen during their consultation with you and which they did not feel able to ask. This often occurs as the patient can feel inhibited and in awe of the dentist.

Many practices offer complimentary appointments with the patient co-ordinator as a precursor to a full consultation with the dentist. This can be particularly beneficial for very nervous patients or for patients who are interested in cosmetic solutions.

Patients are much more likely to discuss treatment options and how they would prefer to finance that treatment when sitting comfortably in a private area within the practice. Provided he or she is adequately trained, the co-ordinator will be able to explain benefits of the proposed plan and arrange the most suitable method of payment; for example, an interest-free payment plan. This means the completion of paperwork associated with financing treatment and making appointments for treatment can be completed outside of the surgery environment, leaving the dentist free to practice dentistry.

If you offer a monthly patient plan at the practice, the patient co-ordinator has the ideal opportunity to fully explain the benefits of the plan to each new patient. Revenue received by direct debit from patients to cover their check ups, hygiene treatments and other benefits is a valuable and predicable source of income for your business. Having a large number of patients registered at the practice on a scheme like this helps to stabilise your private patient list. In order to maximise the advantage of your practice patient plan, you need to be proactive in selling its benefits to your patients, and again this is an area where a patient co-ordinator can add real value to your business.

The role also provides a point of contact at the practice for patients so they may continue to benefit from access to support and advice throughout their treatment in addition to their regular contact with the dentist. The co-ordinator should also be made responsible for tracking all new patients registering at the practice, ensuring they have received all the information they need and that their appointments for treatment are booked before they leave the practice.

The role works particularly well if you have a small room or area that can be converted into a consultation room. The co-ordinator can use visual aids such as models, 'before' and 'after' photographs and DVDs to show patients how proposed treatment will work and provide examples of similar treatments illustrating end results.

In conclusion, I would always recommend that every internal marketing opportunity be exhausted before investing in external marketing. Be sure you and your team are making the most of your existing patients through effective verbal and written communication before trying to generate more business by means of expensive external marketing initiatives.

Direct-debit plan

If you have a monthly direct-debit plan, ensure the patient is provided with a leaflet explaining how the plan works. You may also ask your reception team to inform the patient that 'Dr Smith recommends all his patients join this scheme.' One of the most effective methods to build regular, predictable income for your business is to register as many patients as possible on a monthly direct-debit plan. There are a number of companies who can administer the scheme for you if you prefer not to handle the collection of direct debits at the practice. There are various costs involved relating to the collection of the direct debit, accident and emergency insurance (if desired) and the administration charge.

There are generally two types of plan you can offer your patients: capitation schemes or maintenance schemes. A capitation scheme is based on patients being dentally fit prior to registering on the scheme and then being banded according to the amount of existing dental restoration. The patient then pays a fee per month that covers the cost of their check-ups, hygiene appointments and general dental treatment. Maintenance schemes provide for the costs of check-ups and hygiene appointments only. Patients do not have to be dentally fit to enter the scheme and because of the nature of the scheme, the monthly fees are generally much lower.

Capitation schemes can cost your business a great deal in terms of profit and goodwill if they are not effectively managed. It is imperative to band the patient correctly to begin with and to continue to monitor the dental treatment being received by each patient to ensure they are re-banded when necessary. The practice manager should also carry out checks to ensure patients are only receiving the correct number of hygiene appointments that they are entitled to. In a practice with associate dentists it is advisable to conduct regular audits to ensure supervised neglect is not an issue. Any occurrence of this will damage the goodwill of your business when you come to sell it.

Maintenance schemes are much easier to control as the banding only reflects the number of check-ups and hygiene appointments that patient is to receive in a year. Dental treatment is paid for, sometimes at a discounted rate, so there is no danger of supervised neglect or patients receiving more dental treatment than they are paying for. The practice manager should still conduct audits to confirm patients are only receiving the correct number of hygiene appointments as this, too, will erode profit from a practice, often without the practice owner realising it.

The introduction of a practice maintenance scheme is an ideal mechanism to use to convert a practice to private and is an extremely effective way of retaining a private database of patients. Income received each month is predictable, providing healthy cash flow even when an associate is away from the business.

Interest-free credit

I believe it is important to be able to offer patients the option of spreading the cost of their dental treatment by means of interest-free credit. We live in societies where people rely heavily on being able to purchase the things they want on credit, and dentistry is no different. Some practices now also offer interest-bearing credit to patients who want to spread the cost over longer periods of time.

Being able to offer interest-free or interest-bearing credit will benefit the business in a number of ways. If a practice operates a 'pay-as-you-go' system of collecting fees as and when each part of the patient's treatment is completed, the total fee for the treatment will not be collected until the treatment comes to an end. On the other hand, companies that provide the credit will pay the practice the full amount, less the subsidy charge, as soon as the application for credit has been approved. This improves the cash flow into the business and removes the need to collect a fee from the patient each time they visit the practice. In addition, offering credit to patients allows greater access for patients to choose the dental treatment they want but perhaps cannot afford to pay for immediately, thereby increasing take-up of treatment.

Subsidy rates charged by companies that provide the credit vary and usually increase as the term of the loan is extended. Before making a decision about the company that is right for you, consider the additional benefits of the training and support that some offer to ensure your practice team is marketing the service to patients correctly. Some dentists take a view that the substantial increase in the take-up of treatment offsets the subsidy costs, whilst others increase fees to compensate for the subsidy costs.

To offer interest-free credit, your practice will need to apply for a Consumer Credit Licence, and note that it is illegal to offer the treatment at a lower price for cash, since this discredits the basis upon which the interest-free credit was offered.

CHAPTER 12

Creating a brand identity

When you are in a position to commence external marketing activities, you will need to ensure your business has an identity and brand that will help you develop the profile of your business within the local area.

As a dental professional you should not feel inhibited about developing a strong brand identity and using that identity to illustrate to your local consumer market place why your products and services are best. Provided you supply a clear brief to your graphic design supplier, you should have no fear of undermining your professional dignity.

Once you have your brand identity created, you can then think about commissioning a livery of stationery and informative brochures for your patients and producing a web site for internet enquiries. All your marketing activity, in fact, anything that is customer facing, should be branded so that you develop a consistent and recognisable image that will help your marketing initiatives to gain maximum exposure and results.

Your brand identity needs to say something about you and your business and it should represent the essence of your vision.

It is important that the graphic design company you select to create your brand and logo understands your business and the image you are trying to project. Invite them to the practice for an informal fact-finding meeting. The more information you can provide at this stage, the more likely it is that they will be able to create the kind of image you are looking for. If you are planning to develop the business and offer more private and cosmetic treatment, take this into account when deciding on your logo design. You don't want to have to upgrade the design in a year's time because it no longer represents your business portfolio accurately.

Many designers will base their creative ideas around the name of your practice, so you will need to decide if you are planning to retain this name for your future business or whether the name itself is jaded and old fashioned. Before your meeting with the design team, think about the style you want your identity to portray – classic, contemporary, chic, sophisticated – and think about your target market. To do this, you need to have a good understanding of the demographic profile of your local community so you know the distribution of wealth and social profile of consumers in the vicinity of the practice. This may help you to decide that it's pointless having an ultra-modern chic design aimed at younger members of the local population if the people with disposable income who live locally tend to be in their forties or fifties.

It's also a good idea to decide on a budget for your brand identity, stationery, practice brochure and web site. These costs can escalate and some graphic design companies do not always have a policy of complete transparency on pricing. Ask them to quote for the work that you want doing before you commission them to carry out the task, and make it clear they are not the only company you have invited to tender for the work.

It's difficult to provide a clear idea of costs for you to use as a benchmark and the design fee and printing costs will depend entirely upon the size, quality and quantities of items you ultimately order. However, you could use the following as an approximate guideline:

Logo design and brand identity	£500 to £800
Brochure design	£400 to £1000
Web site design	£1000 to £3000

For this level of investment you can expect a good-quality design job. Of course, you can spend a great deal more, but if this is your first brand identity a reasonably modest investment means the brand can be refined and developed in the future.

It is very difficult to provide a price guide for printing costs for stationery items and promotional leaflets and brochures as the cost will depend upon the quality of paper used, the number of colour processes and the quantity produced. I rarely advise a practice to order more than a thousand of anything unless they know for certain they will consume volume quantities of leaflets, brochures or stationery. Promotional materials such as this can quickly look dated, so keep the quantities reasonably low. Large amounts of stock can also cause storage problems and can become damaged. Provide business cards for well-established associates and have a stock of generic practice cards that can be made available to dental hygienists and newly appointed associates. This will help to keep the costs of design and printing to a minimum.

Another factor to take into account when deciding upon the content of your brochures and leaflets is that you should try to keep references to named people to an absolute minimum. You could consider having a folder instead of a bound patient brochure. This provides a smart and practical loose-leaf holder for individually produced information leaflets that can easily be updated without compromising on the rest of the copy or design. You can even ask your designer and printer to provide a stock of blank leaves printed with your branding which you can use as a template at the practice for one-off leaflets or short-term promotions.

Everything that is visible to the patient has the potential to reinforce your brand identity. Check the quality of all standard letters that are printed and provided to patients as they, too, should be uniform and consistent in font, layout and content.

Once you have received your stock of promotional material and stationery, ensure all the team is fully aware of where this material should be displayed and when promotional items should be handed or posted to patients. Make one person responsible for checking stocks on a regular basis to ensure you can re-order in time for replenishment before the practice runs out. Incorporate usage of your practice literature into the patient experience so that you add another facet of value to their visits to the practice.

Whilst your new brand and literature may look extremely smart, it will only provide a return on investment if you use it to its fullest extent. A pile of leaflets or brochures in reception or tucked into a corner of the surgery will not maximise the opportunity you have to reinforce key messages, educate and inform your patients.

All new private patients should receive a standard letter of welcome, together with a pack of information that will inform them about your practice and the range of products and services on offer. You may wish to include a medical history form for completion to save time when the patient visits the practice for the first time.

Once you have succeeded in registering new patients it is important to maintain effective communication with them. You can use your patient recall system as a means of informing your patients of new products, services and offers. Instead of sending a standard letter to recall each patient, you can incorporate an offer with a closing date to encourage patients to make their recall appointment promptly. Or consider replacing the standard letter altogether, using instead a recall card which can incorporate a voucher or some information on one side and an appointment card on the other, providing a convenient place for the patient to note the appointment date and time when they contact the practice.

Internal newsletters are a good method of communicating with patients, particularly when there have been several developments or changes at the practice that existing patients may not be aware of. This could include a practice refurbishment, the introduction of a new piece of technology, or news about the team. Patients do feel valued each time you communicate with them and even something as straightforward as a recall should be seen as a marketing opportunity.

Establish and monitor your referral source

It is vitally important to know where your new patients are learning about your practice, particularly if you are planning to invest in marketing. At the end of each month you will want to have this useful information at your disposal so you can judge the most and least productive areas of marketing activity. Some computerised patient management systems have a 'referral source' field on the 'patient details' screen. The reception team need to be briefed on the importance of not only filling this field in but also entering the correct referral source details. This field can be set as a mandatory field to encourage your team to fill it in each and every time.

Your practice manager should check this report regularly as it provides critical information about where your new patients hear about you. It will become an even more important source of information when you start investing in external marketing so you can establish the return on the investment you have made in promotional activity. Your practice manager will also need to update the referral sources to include specific promotional activities to ensure the data continues to be accurately recorded and reported.

For example, a typical referral source list may include:

➤ word of mouth referral
➤ named patient referral
➤ Yellow pages
➤ Thomson directory
➤ internet
➤ walked by the practice
➤ open event advertisement
➤ radio advertising campaign.

If you do not have the luxury of a computerised patient management system that shows a referral source field, keep a book at reception and instruct the reception team to retain a written record. This record can be developed further as a tracking document recording when the patient registers and proceeds through to treatment. It will help you to measure the true value of marketing in terms of financial return.

You may also want to introduce a method of recognising those patients who have referred friends and family to the practice. This could be something as simple as a letter of thanks from the principal dentist to a more tangible token of your appreciation such as flowers or champagne.

TABLE 12.1 Example – new patient tracking report

Patient name and DOB	Referral source	Cons	Hyg	Tx	Total value
Tom Bailey 4.7.61	Yellow Pages	1.1.07	7.1.07	14.1.07	3000 IF*
John Arnold 28.10.38	word of mouth	1.1.07	3.1.07	no	450
Susan York 1.3.74	wedding show	3.1.07	14.1.07	22.1. 07	4500 IF*
Katie Moore 24.5.86	wedding show	5.1.07	28.1.07	4.2.07	450

*IF Interest-free patient loan

You can develop the number of columns to provide more information, such as the type of treatment completed; however, multiple columns can make the task of completing the tracking report a time-consuming job for your reception team. This tracking form also provides a very useful management tool when managing the performance of the clinicians, as we shall see in Chapter 15.

If you are planning to invest in external marketing initiatives, budgeting is an important factor to consider when developing your marketing plan. It is easy to get carried away with marketing promotions and fail to keep tabs on what you are spending and on whether these additional costs are creating new and profitable business for you.

Once you start an advertising or promotional campaign, you will find it is not only new patients who will be attracted to your business. Be prepared to be inundated with calls from advertising agencies, offering fantastic deals on late available space. Also be very cautious before signing contracts or parting with money and always check on the credentials of any company touting for your business. You will find a number of unscrupulous operators will contact you, purporting to be something they are not. They demand payment up front for the booking of an exciting advertising opportunity and you may never hear from them again.

Planning your marketing strategy

Your marketing plan should be interwoven with the objectives of your business plan. If your business grossed £1m last financial year and you are looking to develop it to gross £1.3m next year, you need to decide how you are going to deliver that growth to the business. This approach will enable you to generate a number of ideas to help you achieve your aims following a logical and well-structured plan.

First of all, review all the marketing and promotional activity carried out previously and assess the value it delivered to your bottom line. Pick out those initiatives that worked well and discard those that proved to be a waste of time and money.

Decide how much of a marketing budget you are going to allow, based on a percentage of your turnover. For example, you may elect to spend 2% of your projected turnover on marketing costs – which in the case of £1.3m turnover would be £26,000. Divide your budget up throughout the year, avoiding holiday periods, into four marketing campaigns.

If you are planning a marketing strategy that requires expenditure, it is important to establish a method to measure the amount of revenue generated from each marketing activity. As previously described, this can be monitored by ensuring your reception team carefully records the correct referral source for each new patient registering. You can then add up the total amount of revenue generated from these patients. Marketing costs have to be funded from profit and not from turnover, so work out the profit from revenue generated through marketing to establish true return on your investment.

Return on investment example

➤ gross profit margin: 50%
➤ investment in marketing: £20,000
➤ new revenue generated from marketing: £45,000
➤ return on investment: £2,500.

In this example, £22,500 (or 50%) of the revenue generated from marketing is profit. The marketing activities cost £20,000 which means the business had a return on its investment in marketing of £2,500.

Once the budget has been set and you are confident all your internal marketing standards are in place, a plan can be drawn up, spreading the budget throughout the forthcoming year.

CHAPTER 13

Maximising external marketing opportunities

One of the most cost-effective places to carry your brand outside your practice is the pavement in front of your premises. A free-standing advertising board will generate a great deal of interest from passing traffic, particularly if you keep the information fresh by changing the posters regularly. You may need to seek permission from your local council to display an advertising board, so check with them first before purchasing one.

The type of information to consider displaying on an advertising board could include:

➤ open events
➤ free cosmetic consultations
➤ patient schemes
➤ seasonal offers, such as tooth whitening or a free electric toothbrush with every new consultation.

Another simple and cost-effective method of marketing outside your practice is to fix Perspex leaflet holders on the outside of your building. You may be surprised how many passers-by will take a leaflet if they don't have to cross the threshold. It's a very effective way of providing information about your practice and to encourage new enquiries.

Advertising in directories can be effective, particularly if the area your practice is located in has a transient or growing population, as this can be directly related to how many people will search for a new dentist when moving to the area. Review the quantity, size and quality of existing dental practice adverts before designing your own. Colour adverts are considerably more expensive, but do have the advantage of providing greater impact to your advert. Think carefully about the wording of your advert. You may wish to place more emphasis on the features and benefits of your practice that will attract the type of individual who would be using a directory such as the Yellow Pages to find a dentist. For example, you could focus on the fact that you offer quality general dentistry for all of the family, if your practice was located in a region where there was a lot of housing development in progress.

Patients seeking cosmetic options are more likely to search on the internet than in a directory and you will want to provide your web designer with key words that will help to optimise your position within search engines.

If you are considering an advertising campaign, choose the magazine or newspaper that your target market reads. Publications will be able to provide you with information about the demographic profile of their readers to help you choose the right one for your campaign. You will be able to negotiate a discount for multiple bookings and may be able to upgrade the position of your advertisements to maximise their visibility and impact. Try to secure space on the right side of the page as this provides an ideal position for readers to notice your advert. Banners top or bottom can also be very effective. Before you book the space, agree on the price, based on full colour and including any necessary artwork. You will find the impact of advertising is maximised by having a series of advertisements rather than just one big one. The content of the advert can simply communicate your presence and develop brand awareness, or you may want to provide a 'call to action' – in other words, a message that motivates the reader to contact the practice. This may take the form of an open event or a promotional offer.

Open events can be very effective if you have a new product or service to introduce. A smile makeover open event could provide an ideal opportunity to introduce tooth whitening, dental implants and cosmetic dentistry options such as Invisalign to new and existing patients. You can promote the event to existing patients by enclosing invitations within the monthly recall run and externally by placing two to three adverts in the local paper in the weeks running up to the event. The communication of the full range of treatments you offer at the practice to your existing patient database is very important. Patients who have been registered at a practice for many years have been known to go to an alternative practice for cosmetic treatment because they did not realise their own dentist carried out the treatment they wanted.

Competitions can also be a very effective way of developing the profile of the practice. Approach your local newspapers to see whether they would be interested in running competitions. Some are keen to give editorial space free on the basis that competitions are a healthy means of maintaining their readership. You may find some will want an advertising fee for the competition details but will then cover the results with a report and photograph of the winner. Prizes can be anything from an electric toothbrush to five readers; tooth whitening, or a smile makeover worth £5000. Some practices have found that offering the chance to enter a prize draw to win a smile makeover is a very effective way to encourage people to attend open events. This also provides a good PR opportunity – provided the patient has given written permission to allow publicity.

Any event or development of your service should be seen as potential PR and newspapers will cover stories provided they deem them to be newsworthy. For example, your practice may have an adopted charity that your team raises funds for throughout the year, and this is just the sort of story a local newspaper would be willing to run. The practice may have invested in some new state-of-the-art technology or have a member of the team who has done something extraordinary outside of the practice.

Every contact with existing patients represents a marketing opportunity and an important part of your marketing strategy should incorporate plans to communicate with them on a regular basis. It is much more difficult to win new patients than it is to influence the choices your existing patients make about their dental treatment.

Before planning an external marketing campaign, review the quality of customer service and the standard of care your new 'customers' are going to receive. Investment in marketing at the wrong time can be costly if the experience you provide to new patients is not exceptional. When you are confident they will be delighted with the treatment and service they will receive, you can invest in marketing and be sure for every new patient you win, you will grow your business organically from the word-of-mouth referrals that occur as a result of their experience.

SECTION 4

Quality management systems and procedures – Processes underpin your business

---

'Quality is never an accident; it is always the result of high intention, sincere effort, intelligent direction and skilful execution; it represents the wise choice of many alternatives.'

WILLIAM A. FOSTER

Introduction

The content of this book so far has focused on the importance of developing and managing the team that is going to provide quality care and service to your patients, and on the impact that internal and external marketing can have upon your business.

Interwoven with these critical factors are the systems and procedures your business will need to have in place in order to support the quality of service you deliver. Patient complaints can often occur due to a weakness in a system rather than as a result of poor customer service, poor treatment or inadequate training. Additionally, there is an ever-growing number of legal and statutory requirements that must be followed and the practice management must be able to provide evidence of compliance with these.

Clinical Governance was introduced to the profession in the UK by the GDC to encourage dental practice owners to develop a formal and documented approach to patient care and to maintain quality standards within the profession. The requirements of Clinical Governance – which is a quality management system in its own right – are:

➤ a system to ensure that all dental care provided is of a consistent quality
➤ a system to ensure that effective measures of infection control are used
➤ a system to ensure that all legal requirements for Health and Safety are satisfied
➤ a system to ensure that all legal requirements relating to radiological protection are satisfied
➤ a system to ensure that any requirements of the General Dental Council in respect of the Continuing Professional Development of dentists are satisfied.

In addition to these requirements, there are the more practical aspects of running a practice that need to be planned and mapped out to ensure quality standards are being achieved. A lack of clear policies and procedures can lead to poor communication and errors occurring, which can damage the relationship you have with your patients and cost your business profit and lost time.

For example, a practice that has a haphazard approach to the control of laboratory work with no process to manage collection, tracking and delivery of items will almost certainly experience occasions when the patient has an appointment which requires laboratory work to complete the procedure, but the work is still at the dental laboratory. The appointment has to be postponed, annoying both patient and dentist, and costing the business time and money.

The mapping of the processes required to deliver the end product to the patient is an intrinsic factor in the efficient and predictable running of your operation. All processes, systems and procedures should be incorporated into a practice management manual so that the team has a central reference point whenever they need it and new staff can be trained using the contents of the manual as standard.

CHAPTER 14

Practice management manual

There are various generic manuals available which form the basis of many of the legal and standard procedures required to be carried out within a dental business. The final section of the manual will be made up of your practice-specific procedures that help your business to run smoothly.

A good way to decide whether you need to document a procedure is to carry out an audit. Ask your team to log any errors or problems that may have an impact on the quality of care and service you provide to your patients. At the end of the audit period, review the log and collate the results to help identify weaknesses in your operation.

New processes can then be mapped for each procedure that has had an entry in the error log, providing work instructions for the team to ensure that the chance of the same error being repeated is minimised. You can then introduce a continuous cycle of audit to check whether the procedure is still being correctly followed and to implement any changes required.

The control of documents and updates is an important consideration when maintaining a manual. To note each update in chronological order, use the simple method of numbering each new document as the next version. So an amend to Petty Cash procedure V1.0 would become V1.1, making it easy to keep track of changes and the most up-to-date version.

It is not possible to illustrate all the standard operating procedures required to run a dental practice effectively within the scope of this publication. A number of documents have been selected to provide examples of policies, standard operating procedures and audits and risk assessments for your information.

Case studies of practice management processes relating to patient systems

Managing patient debt

Case study

I came across a practice that had accumulated debt of nearly 200k. This major financial problem had been allowed to occur because accounts for services rendered were posted to patients following their treatment and there was no process to chase the accounts.

Clearly the situation could not be allowed to continue and overnight we implemented a new policy of 'pay as you go' for patients. This needed careful and sensitive management by staff at the front desk and they needed lots of encouragement and support to follow the new practice policy, particularly for the first few weeks. Once the staff realised the magnitude of the problem, they were committed to recovering the debt, and at the last count the debt stood at under 10k.

Patient debt can build up to a considerable level if allowed to do so and the recovery of debt can be a time-consuming and sometimes not very pleasant task. It is wise, therefore, to have a systematic approach to the collection of monies to ensure patients do not leave the practice without paying for the treatment they have received.

The most important aspect of managing debt is to ensure systems and procedures are in place to prevent debt from occurring in the first instance.

When debt is allowed to remain unpaid for a long period of time, the prospect of debt recovery reduces considerably and there is an impact on the profit of the practice, caused by the costs in time to recover debt and fees charged by debt-recovery agencies.

Process

1. Create the right culture within your team. Hold a briefing, inform them of the amount of outstanding debt. Remind associates and hygienists they only get paid on monies received and not on invoiced treatments. They have a part to play in ensuring patients pay each time they visit the practice.
2. Ensure patients are accompanied back to reception and that the invoice from work completed that day is produced without unnecessary delay. If notes are still being written up, the clinician should still be able to confirm the amount due today so the payment can proceed. Not only is this good customer service, but it also prevents patients from slipping out the door without paying.
3. Review the content of your patient literature. Do you have a clearly stated policy on payment? Are your patients aware of the policy? The example below shows how your policy can be communicated in a positive way.

Example

OUR COMMITMENT TO YOU

➤ We will listen carefully to your concerns about your dental needs.

➤ We will provide quality dentistry in safe and comfortable surroundings.

➤ We will always be friendly and helpful.

YOUR COMMITMENT TO US

➤ We ask you to attend all the appointments you have made with us or provide at least 24 hours' notice of cancellation when necessary.

➤ We ask you to take care of your oral health and use the maintenance techniques we teach you.

➤ We ask you to settle your fees upon request.

➤ If you are happy with the treatment and service we provide, please refer patients you feel would also benefit from the services we offer.

1. Carry out team training so your front-of-house staff can confidently deal with requesting for payment and overcome objections or excuses.

2. When a patient consents to go ahead with treatment, use this as an opportunity to establish how they intend to finance their treatment. Some practices split the cost over the number of appointments required in order to help spread the cost for the patient, so instead of one large bill being presented at the end of treatment when all the work has been completed, the patient may pay, say, £200 per appointment. Or offer the interest-free payment scheme. This is an ideal method of dealing with debt as the payment is made by the lender, less any subsidy payment, at the start of the treatment. Cash flow of the business benefits and the front-of-house team doesn't have to ask for payment each time the patient comes to the practice.

3. Consider taking deposits to cover the cost of sale items such as laboratory or implant components.

4. Always take monies in advance for tooth whitening.

5. Make one nominated person at the practice responsible for monitoring debt and sending out debt-recovery letters.

6. Use the patient debtor report if available to run off debt for the practice as a whole and for each clinician. This will help focus the clinical team on the part they play.

7. Don't continue with a treatment plan if the patient is in debt. Make suitable financial arrangements with the patient to help them pay off the debt before proceeding.

8. Use standard letters and techniques for debt recovery following a set time frame to ensure the debt is recovered as quickly as possible.

Some sample standards letters have been provided; however, you should rarely need to use them if you follow the steps set out above.

LETTER 1 (SENT WITHIN 3 WORKING DAYS)

Dear Mrs Bailey

It was a pleasure to see you at the practice recently for your dental appointment.

I have enclosed a statement of account for your convenience, showing the fee now due for payment.

You may wish to send a cheque made out to The Dental Practice at the practice address or you may prefer to pay using your debit or credit card by telephoning the practice. We will quickly deal with your payment and send you a receipt in the post. One of our team will contact you shortly to confirm your preferred method of payment.

I look forward to seeing you again at your next appointment.

Yours sincerely

Treating clinician

LETTER 2 (SENT 10 WORKING DAYS FROM DATE OF LETTER 1)

Dear Mrs Bailey

Reference: Fee overdue for dental services received £XXXX

I wrote to you on the xxxxxxx enclosing a statement of account relating to your appointment on the xxxxxxx. I understand from your records that payment has not been received for this appointment and that practice staff have not been able to reach you by telephone.

I know you, as a valued patient, are aware of our policy on payment of dental services received and I would be grateful if you would contact the practice without delay to settle the outstanding amount. If you have any difficulty in making payment please contact the practice manager who will be able to discuss and agree suitable financial arrangements with you.

Thank you for your co operation in this matter.

Yours sincerely

Treating clinician

LETTER 3 (SENT 10 WORKING DAYS FROM DATE OF LETTER 2)

Dear Mrs Bailey

Reference: Fee overdue for dental services received £XXXX

According to my records, there remains an amount unpaid for dental services I provided to you on the xxxxxxxx.

Unfortunately you have not contacted the practice to discuss this outstanding fee and although we have tried repeatedly to call you we have been unable to speak to you regarding this matter.

I feel I have no alternative other than to instruct an agency that specialises in the recovery of debt to contact you on my behalf. I wish to avoid this action at all costs as your credit rating will be affected by this measure.

I will therefore delay this action by three working days only to allow sufficient time for you to contact the practice to arrange payment.

Please contact my practice manager today to arrange settlement to avoid this action.

Yours sincerely,

Treating clinician

The building up of debt within the practice can also disguise cash discrepancies. The security of cash at your reception desk can be compromised when a debt remains on the patient's account for a long time. Dishonesty amongst staff is a rare but existing problem in all businesses. I have found some staff taking advantage of poor cash management and the issue is only revealed when the recovery of debt is made a priority. Many patients who have an aged debt on their account maintain they paid in cash at the time of the visit. There is no record of the cash payment having been made, however, so either the patient is confused about the payment or the cash did not make it into your cash box. If, however, you have a proactive approach to minimising and recovering debt, there is less opportunity for someone to take advantage of the situation as the number of patients owing money will be small and the amounts will not be very old.

One issue you may face if your practice does need to tighten up on debt control is in dealing with patients who have been used to a culture where it is acceptable to leave the practice without paying. To help staff manage and overcome patients' objections, they may need training to develop their levels of confidence in dealing with unhappy patients. This will help them to address the issue and then control it in the future. It's also a good idea to ask your practice manager to report debt levels to you on a weekly basis to ensure you and your manager are focused on constantly monitoring debt levels within your business. If you have had issues in this area and have allowed debt to accumulate, it will take time to recover the monies owed to you. However, this should be a short-term additional commitment for your front-of-house team. You may also have to take the decision to write some of the debt off. If patients have moved away from the address held on your system you will have very little chance of recovering the money that is owed by them.

'Fail to attend' and late cancellations

Case study

During one practice health check, I asked the practice owner if patients failing to attend dental appointments was a problem. The practice team had never measured the cost of this common problem and the practice owner was astounded when the cost was totalled at over 32k in one year.

Patients who habitually fail to attend appointments or cancel at late notice represent a huge cost to practice business in wasted time and lost revenue. A consistent approach to patients ensures that a culture is developed where it is not acceptable to fail to attend appointments or to cancel at late notice.

Practice managers should ensure that 'fail to attend' and late cancellation appointments are monitored and managed to keep them to a minimal level. The number and cost of appointments lost in this way should be included in the management report each month (discussed in next section).

Process

1. Courtesy calls should be made to all patients 48 hours prior to their appointment to confirm the appointment day and time, or a text messaging service can be set up on many patient management systems.
2. If a patient fails to attend, a nominated member of staff, i.e. nurse or hygienist must call the patient and express concern that they have not attended their scheduled appointment, using the following wording, 'Mrs Brown, this is Anywhere Dental practice, we were concerned that you failed to attend your appointment with Dr Green today, is there a problem?'
3. The practice manager must use their knowledge of the patient and their common sense before deciding what course of action to take. Take into account:
   — whether the patient has failed to attend previously
   — whether they are loyal patients
   — what the circumstances were that caused the failure to attend the appointment.
4. Patients can be encouraged to guarantee their appointment with a deposit or paying up front, using the following wording, 'Mrs Brown, I have booked your appointment with Dr Green. As we have ordered materials especially for your treatment on that day, he has asked that you place a deposit with us to cover the cost of the materials and secure that appointment.'
5. Or, 'Mrs Brown, I know you are very busy so if you would like to settle your hygiene appointment in advance it will save you time when you attend.'

There are many different ways of phrasing requests like this in a positive and constructive way. Do not be put off by the occasional negative comment by patients and be prepared to offer a reasonable explanation to counter their objections:

'Mrs Brown, I do understand that you feel reluctant to pay in advance for your treatment. Some of our other patients have felt that way too. When we explain that it helps us to prepare in advance for your appointment, most of our patients have found that to be quite acceptable.'

You need to get the whole team on board with this policy as the message can be reinforced throughout the practice. Encourage patients to pay in advance or by large instalments – particularly for long appointments. This is particularly important if the appointment involves an anaesthetist as you will incur cost once their services are booked, whether or not the patient attends.

You will find that adopting this approach creates a culture where patients do not fail to attend appointments as they value the service and time you are dedicating to them as individuals.

You may 'lose' a few disgruntled patients who are habitual 'fail to attend' clients or cancellers – these patients are costing your business time and money so be prepared to let them go.

Informed patient consent

Case study

I was recently made aware of a very unfortunate situation where a patient complained to the GDC because the course of their treatment was altered once it had commenced and the dentist had not sought ongoing consent from the patient for the changes in his treatment which would have cost the patient an additional fee.

This dentist is an excellent practitioner whose only error was not to record the explained changes in treatment and cost for the patient. When the patient was asked to pay, he claimed he have never given his consent for the treatment plan to change. His complaint was upheld by the GDC and the dentist was reprimanded.

This is one important area that sometimes gets overlooked and clinicians leave themselves at risk of complaints from patients and a reprimand from the GDC. The agreement to carry out treatment and the cost of that treatment needs to be absolutely clear from the outset to avoid misunderstandings. Complaints relating to informed consent often occur when the treatment that has been planned has to be changed. For example, if a simple extraction turns into a surgical extraction, the clinician should discuss the implications of this with the patient in terms of risks, benefits, costs and alternatives before proceeding with treatment.

Patients have a basic legal right to receive appropriate information before they consent to examination, treatment or care. Seeking consent and recording it in the patient's notes protects both the patient and the clinician and should ensure that patients can give their consent for treatment based on information that communicates the benefits, risks, options and alternatives involved with that proposed treatment.

The practice manager is responsible for ensuring the procedure for informed patient consent is designed, implemented and maintained within the quality systems and procedures.

Clinicians are responsible for ensuring that informed consent is sought from patients and recorded in the patient notes. Consent is ongoing and clinicians are responsible for ensuring their patients are kept informed at each stage of their examination, treatment and care. Gaining consent is a process and not a one-off event, and patients can withdraw their consent at any time. It is best practice for the person actually treating the patient to seek the patient's consent. Consent may be sought on behalf of colleagues only if *the person seeking consent is capable of carrying out the treatment, or has had special training to seek consent for that procedure.*

➤ Patients have given implied consent to be examined through the process of making an initial appointment. Patient consent for the clinician to carry out

X-rays, treatment and any other diagnostic procedures must be confirmed verbally. It is the clinician's responsibility to do this.

➤ Adults are always assumed to be competent unless demonstrated otherwise. Ask yourself, 'Can this patient understand and weigh up the information needed to make this decision?' Unexpected decisions may not indicate incompetence, only that the patient requires further information or explanation.

➤ Patients may be competent to make some healthcare decisions but not others.

➤ Giving and obtaining consent is not a one-off event. Patients can change their mind and withdraw consent at any time. If in doubt, the clinician must check that the patient still consents to be cared for or treated.

Consent and children

➤ You must seek consent before examining, treating or caring for children.

➤ Young people aged 16 and 17 are presumed to have the competence to give consent for themselves.

➤ Younger children who fully understand what is involved in their proposed treatment can also give consent.

➤ In other cases, someone with parental responsibility must give consent on the child's behalf.

➤ If a competent child consents to treatment then a parent cannot override that consent.

➤ Legally, a parent can consent if a competent child refuses, but it is unlikely that this serious step would be taken.

Informed consent in adults

➤ Patients require sufficient information before they can decide whether to give consent; for example, they must have information about the benefits, costs, and risks of the proposed treatment, and about alternative treatments.

➤ A patient's consent may not be valid if they have not been offered as much information as they may reasonably require in order to make their decision.

➤ Consent must be given voluntarily and not under any form of duress or undue influence from health professionals, family or friends.

➤ Consent may be obtained in writing, verbally or non-verbally. A signature on a consent form does not itself prove the consent is valid – the point of the form is to record the patient's decision, and also, increasingly, the discussions that have taken place.

➤ The clinician is required to seek consent from the patient prior to initial examination and prior to treatments carried out on that patient. Consent to continue to care for that patient must be sought at every subsequent examination.

➤ Competent adults can refuse treatment even where it would clearly benefit their health.

➤ No one can give consent on behalf of an incompetent adult. You may still treat this patient if the treatment would be in the best interests of the patient. These interests extend beyond medical interests and can include factors such as the wishes and beliefs of the patient when they were competent, to their overall well-being and spiritual and religious welfare. Where a patient has never been competent, relatives and carers may be best placed to advise on the patient's needs and preferences. If an incompetent patient has clearly indicated in the past, while competent, that they would refuse treatment (an advance refusal) and those circumstances arise, you must abide by that refusal.

➤ Signed consent forms must be retained in the patient file for future reference.

Example: Consent form

PATIENT CONSENT FORM

Please take a few moments to consider whether we have provided you with sufficient information and, where necessary, explanation to enable you to give informed consent regarding your treatment or care at Anywhere Dental Care. We want you to understand the benefits of receiving treatment from us, any risks associated with that treatment and what other options may be available to you. We want you to have the confidence that you are being offered a consistent standard of care and treatment and that all aspects of your treatment are fully discussed with you.

Financing of the cost of your proposed treatment may be discussed with our practice manager as we have a number of options available for you to consider.

Please ask a member of our team for further explanation if required.

TABLE 14.1 Informed consent form

Patient's name:
Patient's date of birth:
Patient's address:
Type of treatment:
Estimated cost of treatment:
I have been given the necessary information about and explanation of my proposed treatment, the risks, benefits and any alternatives and its costs and hereby give my informed consent for the treatment to continue.
Signed...
Dated ....

Archiving and storage of patient records

The storage and archiving of all records, particularly patient records, is an important responsibility for practice owners. Whether the records are computer records or paper-based records, they must be kept in secure conditions to protect the confidentiality of the patient and ensure they are accessible if required.

The practice manager will be responsible for ensuring that all records, files and documents are archived, stored and disposed of following legal requirements and the practice standards.

Process

1. Patient records must be kept for as long as possible and for at least 11 years; and in the case of children, up to age 25 or for 11 years, whichever is the longer. This includes study models and radiographs.
2. Information obtained in the course of dental care is confidential and can only be divulged to third parties, without the patient's consent, under certain limited conditions. These restrictions include the fact that a patient is registered at a practice, has attended the practice or has a future appointment at the practice.
3. Patients have the right of access to their health records held on computer and their manual records.
4. Archived records must be retained in a secure condition that allows authorised access when required.
5. Patient records that can be destroyed must be disposed of securely by shredding or incineration.
6. Paper copies of practice documents relating to the practice management system should be stored for a period of three years with the most recent being the topmost document.
7. All documents archived will be boxed-filed in disposal order with the most recent documentation being held at the front or the top, depending on box-file type. Storage areas for archived material and suitable containers will be practice specific.
8. Final disposal of all paper documents will be dependent upon the level of security which needs to be supplied.
   - Patient records – retain for a minimum of 11 years, then shred.
   - Management information – retain for 3 years, then shred.
   - Practice management system documents – retain for 3 years, then shred.
   - Technical literature – retain until replaced, and then dispose of conventionally.
   - All paper information for disposal must be recycled whenever possible.

Case studies of practice management documents relating to human resource systems

Manual handling

Case study

Musculoskeletal injury from poor posture, poor lifting and wear and tear leads to millions of working days lost in the UK and can lead to long-term chronic conditions and affect capacity to work.

This problems can manifest themselves in something as apparently innocuous as a stiff neck, to a sudden, acute injury sustained through an accidental injury.

When I asked one practice owner if he had a manual handling policy, he showed me a full set of instructions and up-to-date record cards to show that all his staff and clinicians had received full manual handling training and instruction.

The reason for his careful attention to detail was an accident that had occurred in his practice the previous year, when a dental nurse had lifted a water bottle in completely the wrong way, seriously injuring her back. Whilst she did make a recovery, she continues to suffer the long-term effects of the injury.

Practice owners have a duty of care to provide patients, visitors, employees and associates with a safe working environment and the training and guidance to ensure all activities carried out within the practice are conducted in an appropriate and safe manner. All employees and associates have a personal responsibility to take every reasonable precaution to minimise the risk of injury due to poor posture or manual handling. Millions of working days a year are lost due to injuries sustained at work, many of which are entirely preventable. Procedures to reduce and manage the risk of sustaining injury through poor manual handling must be followed by all associates and employees of the company.

The practice manager is responsible for ensuring all staff and associates are trained in safe manual handling techniques in accordance with the practice policy and procedure. All employees and associates are responsible for following the standard indicated in the practice policy and procedure, thus contributing to a safe working environment at all times and minimising the risk to themselves and others by following the procedures.

Process

1. The practice manager must ensure that all staff and associates working within the practice have received the *Manual Handling Procedure, Work Instruction* and that the *Staff Training Record* is updated accordingly.
2. All new staff induction must include briefing on *Manual Handling Procedure, Work Instruction* and the *Staff Training Record* must be updated accordingly.
3. A *Risk Assessment* must be completed throughout the practice to establish the activities taking place that may increase the risk of a manual handling injury. Upon completion, risks identified must be managed to minimise the possibility of injury occurring.
4. The *Risk Assessment* form must be retained with the *Manual Handling Procedure*

and any remedial action taken must be recorded on a *Corrective and Preventive Action* form, a copy of which must be retained with the *Risk Assessment* form and the *Manual Handling Procedure*.

5. The *Staff Training Record* must be updated with any practice-specific procedures that result from the *Risk Assessment*.

6. Any accidents must be recorded in the *Accident Book* and fully investigated to establish whether any remedial action is necessary. Any recommended action must be recorded, and retained with the *Manual Handling Procedure*. For further information on Health and Safety, please refer to *Health and Safety Policy and Procedures*.

7. Accidents resulting in serious injury or absence from work must be reported to the Health and Safety Executive (HSE).

TABLE 14.2 Manual handling work instruction

Manual handling work instruction
Bend from the knees, keeping back straight to ensure leg muscles take the strain of bending and lifting.
Before attempting to lift an object, assess the overall size and weight. Only objects that are well within an individual's lifting capacity should be lifted.
Place feet on firm, flat surface, shoulder-width apart prior to lifting object, with one foot placed in front of the other.
Lift object at its most rigid point, ensuring the edge of the object is firmly positioned into the palm of the hand with fingers placed to support the weight and balance of the object.
Always hold the object close to your torso – holding it away from your body will place strain on back muscles.
Do not store bulky or heavy objects on shelving any higher than shoulder height.
Do not stack bulky or heavy objects at a height that will compromise the stability of the stack.
Never attempt to lift or move an object that appears heavy or awkward.
Do not attempt to remove heavy or bulky objects from shelves or stacks using step-ladders.
Take particular care with containers holding liquid or shifting contents.
Do not carry objects that prevent you from seeing where you are going.
Do not store objects in corridors, or block fire exits.
Always ask for help.
Always consider your bending and lifting position.

Practice and personal security

Case study

A practice I visited recently was having ongoing issues with patients being abusive to the front-of-house team. The team felt a lack of support from the practice owner because he rarely witnessed the rudeness and aggressive behaviour they did. However, once we implemented clear guidelines and communicated the practice policy on aggression, the majority of issues stopped occurring.

The practice security policy is to ensure that people, stock, cash and other assets are protected to provide a safe working environment and to minimise losses that erode profit margins and affect individuals within our team.

The practice manager is responsible for ensuring that security procedures are followed and monitored. Any non-conformance must be addressed immediately and recorded on a *Corrective and Preventive* form. The practice manager is responsible for the security of the practice and its assets. Security procedures are designed to protect people and profit and non-compliance may result in disciplinary action being taken. Practice teams must ensure that every care is taken to follow security procedures and that every reasonable effort is made to protect people and profit.

Process

1. All team members must read and sign the *Computer Users Protocol* and ensure they understand and comply with all rules regarding the secure use of IT equipment within the business.
2. Practice telephones must not be used for personal calls or Internet connections unless permission is given by the practice manager.
3. Drugs retained on the premises for the treatment of patients must be secured at all times in the drugs cupboard. Under no circumstances may drugs be dispensed to members of staff or associates. The practice manager or nominated responsible nurse will be responsible for ensuring the drugs cabinet is secure and that access is via the designated key holder. Inappropriate use of drugs or drugs left in an insecure location will be considered to be a serious breach of security and may result in disciplinary action being taken.
4. Personal property must by kept within the designated area, either in staff rest areas, lockers or other designated locations within the practice.
5. Stock for resale or use within the practice must not be taken for personal use by any team member.
6. Consumable items must be used prudently, keeping wastage to a minimum.
7. Samples of stock given to the practice remain the property of the practice but can be issued to team members at the practice manager's discretion for training purposes.
8. The accounting of monies prior to banking must be completed in a controlled area, either an office or quiet location with the minimum of interruption.
9. Monies waiting to be banked must be retained in a locked container at all times. Team members should take monies to the bank in twos whenever practically possible. The route taken to reach the bank and the timing of the journey should be varied.
10. Cash taken for dental treatments must be placed immediately in a safe location – either a locked cash box or cash register.
11. For procedures on looking after patient property, please see *Patients Property Procedure*.
12. The practice manager must ensure all keys associated with the practice are retained at the practice and clearly labelled. Wherever possible, a spare set

of keys should be retained. Staff allocated keys must sign for them in the *Key Control Register*.

13. In the event of verbal abuse by a patient, the member of staff should remain calm and professional. Report the incident to the practice manager who will take any appropriate action. This must include a full investigation of the circumstances and may in exceptional circumstances result in the patient being de-registered from the practice. The possibility of the patient being in pain or being very nervous must be taken into account at all times.

14. In the event of aggressive behaviour by a patient, the member of staff should remain calm and professional. Attempts should be made to maintain a safe physical distance from the patient. Attempts should be made to maintain an 'escape route' from the patient if necessary. Attempts should be made to alert another member of staff to the situation. The possibility of the patient being in pain or reacting to the administration of drugs must be taken into account at all times. Every attempt must be made to calm the patient to prevent injury to themself or any member of staff or third party. In extreme circumstances where injury or damage to property appears a real possibility, the police should be alerted. All incidents of this nature must be fully investigated by the practice manager.

15. In the event of verbal abuse by a member of the practice team, the incident should be reported to the practice manager who will complete an investigation, following standards set out in *Team Value Statement*. Disciplinary action may be taken depending on the outcome of this investigation.

16. In the event of aggressive behaviour by a member of the practice team, the incident must be reported to the Practice Manager who will complete an investigation, following standards set out in *Team Values Statement*. Aggressive behaviour by members of the practice team to colleagues or patients will be subject to disciplinary action and may be classed as gross misconduct. For disciplinary policies and procedures refer to the personnel section of the core filing system.

17. In the event of intruders or strangers being discovered within the practice who cannot account for their presence legitimately, members of the practice team must on no account place themselves at personal risk. The stranger must be greeted politely and asked if they require any assistance. If they do not provide a satisfactory response they should be escorted off the premises if this can be achieved in a calm manner and without risk of confrontation. If there are signs of aggression, the member of staff must not pursue the matter but must go immediately to a manager and report the incident. In the event of intruders demanding money or goods, at no time must practice staff place themselves at risk of personal attack or injury to protect company monies or property, although all security rules and precautions must be observed to reduce the risk of this occurring.

18. The security of the practice premises must be protected at all times. Cupboards containing confidential or sensitive information must be secured. External

doors must be checked when closing the practice and the practice alarm system must be set according to supplier's instructions.

19. Keys must be listed on a key register, together with the signature of the team member currently in possession of them. Lost keys must be reported to the practice manager.

Example quality documents relating to clinical systems
Accidents and incidents

All accidents and incidents must be recorded and reported following statutory regulations and risk assessments must be maintained to minimise the opportunity for accidents and incidents to occur so that patients, staff and third parties can enter our practices in safety.

Process

1. The practice manager will ensure a quality procedure for accidents and incidents is designed and implemented with the quality manual. The quality procedure will be reviewed as part of internal audit and management review to ensure it continues to meet the needs of the practice.

2. Practice managers are responsible for ensuring all reasonable steps are taken to reduce and manage the risks of accidents and incidents occurring. They are also responsible for staff training and ensuring that all documents are correctly completed and maintained.

3. Practice teams are responsible for taking every reasonable precaution to reduce the risk of accidents or incidents. All hazards must be reported to the practice manager immediately and isolated and labelled if possible. Team members are also responsible for completing all necessary documentation to record an accident or incident.

4. All dental practices must comply with the Reporting of Injuries, Diseases and Dangerous Occurrences Regulation (RIDDOR). The regulations affect dental practices in one of two ways – if an accident occurs at work or if an employee contracts a disease as a result of work.

5. All accidents and incidents must be reported in the accident and incident book, regardless of how minor they are. There must be a written record of the date of the accident, the nature of the injury sustained, where it took place and the circumstances leading to the accident. The name, address and occupation of the person involved in the accident must also be recorded in the accident book.

6. An accident which causes an employee to be absent from work for more than three days must be notified to the Health and Safety Executive within seven days using the HSE 2508 form.

7. Major accidents that involve death, a serious injury such as a broken limb, loss of an eye or admission to hospital for more than 24 hours, must be reported to the Health and Safety Executive at once by telephone. The HSE 2508 form will then need to be completed within seven days of the accident occurring.

8. For procedure to deal with a needle stick injury refer to *Needle Stick Injury* procedure.
9. All notifiable diseases and dangerous occurrences relating to the practice must also be notified to the local Health and Safety Executive.

Control of substances hazardous to health

Example of audit document

Practice name. . . . .
Name of person completing audit . . . .
Position in practice, e.g. manager . . . .
Date audit completed . . . .
Audit to be completed by (date) . . . .

CONTROL OF SUBSTANCES HAZARDOUS TO HEALTH (COSHH)
The COSHH file and this procedure must be read by every member of the team. A note on the *Staff Training Record Card* must be made.

❏ *Checked for compliance*   ❏ *Identified non-compliance*

Control measures such as storage and use of protective clothing must be adhered to at all times.

❏ *Checked for compliance*   ❏ *Identified non-compliance*

Emergency procedures must be clearly accessible and retained in the COSHH file.

❏ *Checked for compliance*   ❏ *Identified non-compliance*

An annual COSHH assessment will have to be completed for your practice or work environment. Use the *Risk Assessment Form* to complete your assessment and add additional substances introduced to the work environment.

❏ *Checked for compliance*   ❏ *Identified non-compliance*

Ensure all substances subject to COSHH are stored in the appropriate location.

❏ *Checked for compliance*   ❏ *Identified non-compliance*

Note: Manufacturers' guidance on containers' warning labels indicate the requirement for COSHH. **Note that data sheets containing all the information you need on substances subject to COSSH are available from suppliers.**

❏ *Checked for compliance*   ❏ *Identified non-compliance*

Record all accidents or incidents relating to COSHH.

❏ *Checked for compliance*   ❏ *Identified non-compliance*

Make sure all staff are aware of COSHH file and what to do in case of emergency.

☐ *Checked for compliance*   ☐ *Identified non-compliance*

Ensure all third parties are adequately protected, e.g. children.

☐ *Checked for compliance*   ☐ *Identified non-compliance*

A core file for Safety Data Sheets should be retained in the core filing system. All newly purchased products subject to COSHH must be added to core file.

☐ *Checked for compliance*   ☐ *Identified non-compliance*

When completing your assessment, remember damage may be caused by inhalation, contact, ingestion or inoculation.

☐ *Checked for compliance*   ☐ *Identified non-compliance*

Hazardous substances most frequently dealt with in a dental practice are:
➤ disinfectants
➤ mercury
➤ blood and other body fluids
➤ latex
➤ bleach
➤ ethyl chloride
➤ nitrous oxide
➤ etchant gel
➤ hydrogen peroxide
➤ X-ray developer and fixer
➤ tray adhesive
➤ oxygen.

Other hazardous substances such as correction fluid or cleaning materials will have all the required information on the container holding the substance. If the manufacturer's label does not indicate a warning, the substance will not need to be included on your risk assessment.

☐ *Checked for compliance*   ☐ *Identified non-compliance*

When conducting your risk assessment you must consider storage, protective clothing, handling, emergency measures, and waste disposal of hazardous material.

☐ *Checked for compliance*   ☐ *Identified non-compliance*

The following considerations must be taken into account:

The steam from the autoclave may contain chemical vapours and should not be inhaled.

❒ *Checked for compliance*   ❒ *Identified non-compliance*

Keep lids on disinfection baths to prevent vapours becoming an irritant.

❒ *Checked for compliance*   ❒ *Identified non-compliance*

Keep lids on ultrasonic baths to prevent aerosols from dispersing.

❒ *Checked for compliance*   ❒ *Identified non-compliance*

Never allow dental materials to come into contact with the skin or inhale fumes from any dental materials.

❒ *Checked for compliance*   ❒ *Identified non-compliance*

Do not inhale X-ray developing fluid vapours.

❒ *Checked for compliance*   ❒ *Identified non-compliance*

Do not inhale dust that may be thrown into the air from polishing fillings, dentures or teeth.

❒ *Checked for compliance*   ❒ *Identified non-compliance*

Familiarise yourself and your team with all the requirements of infection control.

❒ *Checked for compliance*   ❒ *Identified non-compliance*

Office markers, correction fluids or glue can cause contact or inhalation hazards.

❒ *Checked for compliance*   ❒ *Identified non-compliance*

Cleaners should avoid ingestion of cleaning materials and should wear thick rubber gloves to prevent contact irritation.

❒ *Checked for compliance*   ❒ *Identified non-compliance*

Accidental contact, inhalation, ingestion or inoculation of any substance subject to COSHH must be recorded in the accident book and medical advice sought where necessary.

❒ *Checked for compliance*   ❒ *Identified non-compliance*

WORKING SAFELY WITH FLAMMABLE SUBSTANCES

Ensure flammable liquids or gases are stored and used in a well-ventilated area. This will mean that any vapours given off from a spill or leak will be rapidly dispersed.

❑ *Checked for compliance*   ❑ *Identified non-compliance*

Ensure there are no obvious ignition sources in the storage and handling area.

❑ *Checked for compliance*   ❑ *Identified non-compliance*

Ignition sources can include sparks from electrical equipment, cutting tools, hot surfaces, and open flames from heating equipment. Ensure that there is no smoking in all areas.

❑ *Checked for compliance*   ❑ *Identified non-compliance*

Do not forget sunlight is a source of heat. A glass window may intensify heat during the summer to a considerably high temperature and this has been known to cause aerosol cans to explode.

❑ *Checked for compliance*   ❑ *Identified non-compliance*

Ensure flammable substances are stored in a suitable container and separated from general work and storage areas, ideally separated by a physical barrier, wall or partition.

❑ *Checked for compliance*   ❑ *Identified non-compliance*

Do not store flammable liquids or gases near to combustible materials.

❑ *Checked for compliance*   ❑ *Identified non-compliance*

Example of risk assessment form

RISK ASSESSMENT FORM

Risk assessor . . . .
Location of assessment . . . .
Date of assessment . . . .
Area of risk assessed . . . .

EXAMPLES
➤ manual handling
➤ health and safety
➤ COSHH
➤ display screen equipment
➤ clinical
➤ fire risk.

When completing a risk assessment, the risk assessor should ask themselves the following questions:
➤ Is there a risk?
➤ How can it be minimised?
➤ Are effective measures in place and emergency procedures identified and monitored?
➤ Who is particularly at risk?
➤ Have staff been trained?
➤ Does any external agency need to be involved to advise on risk management?

Risk matrix

Risks which are identified must be categorised as follows:
1. Very low risk – identify and note the risk and any preventive measures.
2. Medium risk – identify and note the risk, preventive measures and actions with appropriate timescales.
3. High risk – identify and note the risk and take immediate corrective action to manage risk.

TABLE 14.3 Risk assessment form

Hazard	Potential danger	Risk	Action	By

Conclusion

You can see from the small sample of documents provided that the provision of a manual containing all the necessary information you and your team will need to run your business safely and effectively is not a simple task.

It is not worth taking risks or cutting corners with Health and Safety, or with statutory requirements, as these regulations are in place to protect your people, your patients and your livelihood. There are many organisations that can assist you in these critical areas, many of which will allow you to download standard procedures and regulations free of charge if you are a member of their organisation.

Although it is not a legal requirement to have the documents that relate to the standard operating procedures of your business, it is still well worth going to the trouble of mapping all of your main processes so your team knows how to perform tasks with the minimum chance of error and maximum efficiency. As you and your practice manager monitor and review the effectiveness of these processes, you will continuously improve and streamline your operation, helping to develop a stress-free working environment.

SECTION 5

Management information and reporting – Key performance indicators and how they can drive your business

---

'In the new economy, information, education, and motivation are everything.'

PRESIDENT BILL CLINTON

Introduction

One method of judging the success of your business is to measure how much cash is being generated. This generally provides you with a good idea of whether your business is solvent. However, there are literally dozens of key performance indicators that can be accessed from your systems and manually from within your business that will provide you with information to help you develop your knowledge of your business and focus your efforts on those areas that are costing you money and those areas that have the potential to generate more revenue and profit for you.

In order to effectively drive your business productivity and profit you need to be able to see the whole picture and not make a judgement based just on how much cash you can take from the business in any given month or year.

The regular provision of management information enables you to address areas of concern and to re-focus your and your team's efforts on achieving your true business potential.

If your practice has a computerised patient management system, you should be able to extract variable amounts of management information from this, depending which system you have. If you are currently relying on manual records, you may need to set up some additional recording systems to gather the information and collate it on a regular basis in order to build your management reports.

CHAPTER 15

Defining and analysing dental business key performance indicators

The following key performance indicators are a sample of some of the main areas that will help you to monitor the performance of your business. By monitoring the information gathered on a regular basis, you will be able to establish trends and identify potential areas of concern that require attention. I have provided a brief definition of each indicator, together with how you could maintain a manual record if you do not already have the functionality of a computerised patient system at your disposal.

I have also provided examples of how you can interpret each key performance indicator separately and in relation to others and how you can use this information to improve your practice revenue and profitability.

Hourly rate

This describes the amount of revenue generated per hour, either by clinician or by the practice. There are two different methods that can be used to measure hourly rate – one is based on revenue generated by hours utilised and the other on revenue generated in total hours available. See the example below for an explanation.

Example of hourly rate measurement

1. Associate Dr B generated £1000 of revenue seeing patients for a total of 5 hours out of a 7-hour session, making his hourly rate £200 when worked out against time spent with patients. This method measures hourly rate on total hours utilised.
2. Associate Dr B generated £1000 of revenue in a 7-hour session, making his hourly rate £142.85. This measures hourly rate on total hours available.

Working out both of these rates is a useful exercise, particularly when the findings are correlated with occupancy percentage of the associate, as we shall see.

If you do not have the means to generate an automatic report from your computer system, you can easily work out the figures manually by taking the total number of hours available to treat patients, the total number of hours utilised by treating patients and the total amount of revenue accrued during that time frame.

A low hourly rate based on hours available needs to be considered alongside occupancy percentage, as a low occupancy rate will naturally have an impact upon the hourly rate. A new associate building his book would understandably have a low hourly rate, not only because of occupancy of the book, but also because he or she will be seeing patients for predominantly routine or new examinations. Monitor the changes in hourly rate of a new associate on a weekly basis for his or her first three months. An improvement in both occupancy and hourly rate during these early stages is a good indication that the associate is identifying and prescribing treatment and that patients are booking appointments to have that treatment. If the hourly rate has stayed very low during this phase, it may mean the new associate lacks the confidence to prescribe restorative treatment or perhaps their ability to communicate effectively with patients needs developing.

Occupancy

There are several ways to work out occupancy percentage.

Practice occupancy

Firstly, consider your practice as a whole and work out the maximum number of hours available to treat patients. To do this, follow the example below.

Example of practice occupancy measurement

Number of surgeries in current use: 3
Number of surgeries not in use: 1
Total number of practice opening hours in a week: 40
4 (surgeries) x 40 hours = 160 hours
Number of associates: 5
Total number of hours associates available to see patients: 112

The occupancy percentage of your practice based on current opening hours and total surgery availability is 70%, i.e. 112 hours divided by 160 = 70% of total capacity.

This is a useful exercise to carry out to help establish the additional potential of your business. This example shows the practice is non-productive for 30% of the time.

Should the practice owner refurbish the surgery not in use? There are a number of factors to take into consideration to establish whether further investment at this stage is required.

➤ Firstly, establish the occupancy of each associate (see below). In a private practice, occupancy should be optimised at around 80–85% as this allows flexibility within the appointment book to accommodate restorative cases and last-minute bookings. If the majority of associates are 80% or more occupied, it would be beneficial to extend the availability of appointments.

➤ Next, review the practice opening hours. Currently the practice is open 8 hours a day, 5 days of the week. There is scope to increase these opening hours to include early-morning, late-evening and Saturday-morning appointments – all very popular sessions with patients. Let us assume the practice could open for an additional 10 hours per week, spread over morning, evening and Saturday mornings, and that an additional £2000 per week (based on £200 per hour) would be generated just by doing this. The only investment required would be in some additional staffing to cover the extra shifts.

➤ Then review the availability of associates within the current and proposed opening hours. Even without extending the opening hours, there are 8 hours of the week which are non-productive because the total availability of the associates is 112 hours, and 3 surgeries running on a 40-hour week provides 120 hours of appointment time. By increasing associate availability by 8 hours or taking on a new part-time associate, an additional £1600 of income could be generated per week.

➤ These initiatives have the potential to add 144k onto practice revenue in a year, based on £200 being generated for 40 weeks of the year. A prudent practice owner may decide to do this first to generate the funds to refurbish the fourth surgery once his or her current availability is fully exploited.

Occupancy of associates

To work out the occupancy percentage of an associate, take the total number of hours he or she is contracted to work a week. Then establish how many hours each week the associates spends seeing patients.

Example

Contract: 30 hours per week

		Occupancy	Running average or trend
Week 1	20 hours	66.66%	66.66%
Week 2	22 hours	73.33%	70.00%
Week 3	26 hours	86.66%	75.55%
Week 4	12 hours*	75.00%	75.47%

*Two days annual leave taken this week – therefore availability for work is reduced by 14 hours to avoid corruption of data.

This occupancy figure for a private practice should run at between 75% and 85%. Week 3 looks high but this may be because the associate completed as much work as possible in this week, knowing two days were going to be lost the following week. It is the overall trend that is important to monitor.

When you have determined the average hourly rate and the occupancy percentage of your associates, comparing them with each other provides further useful information. For example, an associate with a low hourly rate and high occupancy may have a problem accommodating restorative cases that would drive the hourly rate up. Carry out an audit to see what the average completion time of a course of treatment is. It may be the associate has too many patients and may need to offload some of them to a colleague.

Some associates are busy but do not prescribe restorative treatment. In such cases, the appointment book tends to be full of routine examinations and very little treatment appointments.

Another tip is to check that your associates are not carrying out scaling and polishing, which increases occupancy but decreases hourly rate.

In some cases, the prescribing profile of the associate looks healthy, occupancy is high, yet the hourly rate is lower that the practice average. This can sometimes be due to the length of time taken for each procedure, or occasionally you may find the associate is not charging the correct fee for the treatment carried out, or sometimes not charging at all for a variety of short appointments. The impact this can have upon the hourly rate is surprising. The only way to establish whether this is the case is to examine closely a day or even a week of treatment to build up an accurate picture of what is happening.

You may be surprised when conducting this exercise with dental hygienists as one would naturally assume that, since the hourly rate is fixed, it should be the same for all hygienists working in the practice based on hours available. However, it is often the case that the hourly rates differ considerably and this can be for a number of reasons. Close inspection can reveal appointment times that have been extended by the hygienist; patients not charged correctly, or time blocked off without apparent reason. Many dental hygienists now prefer to work with a dental nurse and whilst this should maximise the work rate of the hygienist, the cost of providing a nurse must be built into the fee charged to patients otherwise there will be a negative impact upon your profitability.

Example

A dental hygienist works 35 hours per week over four days at, on average, 80% occupancy level. The hourly rate is charged out at £105 and this is generally made up of three 20-minute appointments of £35 each. She therefore generates £2,940 of income per week. The hygienist is paid at an hourly rate of £30 per hour and therefore costs £1,050 per week.

The gross profit is therefore 64%.

If the hygienist requests a dental nurse to assist her, the cost would be in the region of £315 per week, including employer's NI contribution. This additional cost reduces the gross profit margin to 53.5%.

To recover the gross margin, the hourly rate generated would need to increase to £133 per hour at 80% occupancy.

This would mean the charge to the patient increasing to £44 for a 20-minute appointment just to cover the cost of the dental nurse.

An 80% occupancy level does not justify the requirement of a dental nurse as there should be sufficient time within the working day, since 20% of a full day is almost 2 hours. If the dental hygienist was operating at 100% occupancy on the same hourly rate of £105, she would generate £3,675 of income which would fund a dental nurse.

Having key information to hand such as hourly rate and occupancy really assists you and your practice manager to identify and address performance issues with your clinical team and continuously monitor the financial health of your business.

Conversion rate

Conversion rate is defined by measuring the total number of new patients attending consultations against the total number taking up treatment and being retained at the practice.

We have already established in Section 3 (on marketing) how important it is to track the progress of new patients as they register at the practice and attend their first appointment. The conversion rate of new patients is an extremely important key performance indicator for your business, particularly if you are investing in external marketing initiatives.

An additional useful ratio to measure is the number of enquiries made by callers to reception and the subsequent number of consultation appointments made. The reception team should be encouraged to record the reason for the enquiry even if the caller does not make an appointment, as this will help your practice manager to pinpoint issues relating to the effective communication of availability of products and services to prospective patients. A low conversion ratio would indicate that further training is required.

You will want to be sure every new patient has been referred to the dental hygienist for treatment and that the associate is not carrying out that part of the patient's care, or is not prescribing a scale and polish at all.

Assuming the patient has an appointment to see the dental hygienist, you then need to review what treatment, if any, has been prescribed. This exercise is not purely to ensure your associate's prescribing profile is offering restorative treatment to patients, but also to audit treatment plans to ensure over-prescribing is not taking place.

Provided the patient has made appointments for their course of treatment and you are satisfied with the treatment plan, you can then produce a ratio of new patients to converted patients. Ideally, you should be achieving an average of 80% conversion rate or more. In other words, for every ten new patients attending the practice, eight or more of them should be retained. If the figure is lower than this you will need to carry out an investigation to establish the reasons for this. It could be any one, or a combination, of the following.

➤ Patient is disappointed with service or experience so lacks confidence to come back for treatment.
➤ Dentist has not listened to the needs of the patient.
➤ Dentist has overwhelmed the patient with too much information.
➤ Large amount of treatment required has not been presented in stages.
➤ Different methods of financing treatment have not been discussed.
➤ Dentist cannot close the sale.
➤ Dentist decides to commence treatment on first appointment.*

This is just a small sample of some of the issues that will have a negative impact upon conversion rates. Don't forget to include the total number of initial enquiries when you are working out your practice conversion percentage.

Recall of patients

The success of your recall system is an important element of patient retention. You should be in a position to know exactly how many recalls cards or letters have been sent out each month and how many patients make appointments as a result. This key performance indicator can never be completely accurate as patients will respond over an extended period of time to a reminder to make an appointment. However, the average number of patients returning to the practice following a recall will provide an indication of the 'health' of your patient database.

We know that patients registered with a private practice are not as diligent in attending their routine examination appointments and current information estimates fewer than 60% of your patients will attend a recall when they are scheduled to.

If you are recalling 300 patients per month and on average only 100 of them are responding to your reminder, your recalls are running at 33.33%. Taking into consideration that you are not likely to have many more than 50 new patients registering per month at the practice, your patient database will diminish considerably over a period of time.

There are several different measures you can take to address a shrinking patient database.

1. Try a different method of recalling patients. For example, some practices find they get a much better response if they make the appointment in advance for the patient and send that out in the post. Whilst there are a number of patients who need to rearrange their appointment, very few people fail to attend.
2. Try using a recall card in the form of an appointment card rather than a letter. We all lead increasingly busy lives and if you can make the task of contacting the

---

* Patients like to feel in control of their dental treatment and if they have booked for a consultation expecting to pay a known fee, which then turns into a crown prep, it may well put them off from returning to the practice. Unless the patient has particularly asked for a problem to be addressed on the first consultation, commencing any form of treatment devalues the consultation appointment and leaves the patient feeling uncertain about the potential cost of future appointments.

practice easier for the patient, it will help increase recall numbers.
3. Some practice now using TXT messaging to contact patients. This can work well – canvass your patients to see if they would prefer this method.
4. Adapt your recall cards so that you can incorporate a promotion or call to action. For example, 'Book your appointment before 22 March and receive a free oral hygiene pack when you attend', or, '£50 off tooth whitening when you attend your routine examination before 22 May'.
5. Make the appointment with the patient before they leave the practice and then send a reminder letter to confirm the appointment one week before it is due.

Patient conversion to finance schemes

Dental practice owners have a range of financial services they can offer their patients to help them to spread the cost of their dental treatment.

Schemes such as interest-free credit or monthly patient plans are important drivers of treatment-plan take-up and help to create healthy and predictable cash flow for your business.

Extended credit facilities

There are several suppliers of interest-free and interest-bearing facilities specifically designed for the business of dentistry. The subsidy rates charged to you vary from supplier to supplier, but the majority of them increase the percentage of charge to your business in relation to the term of the loan. In other words, it will cost you less to loan £10,000 over one year than it would over two years.

Although the cost to you is not insignificant, with average subsidy rates ranging from 6% to 17%, there is still a good business case that can be made for introducing this valuable service to your patients:
➤ great accessibility for patients to take up restorative and cosmetic treatment
➤ guaranteed payment of the whole amount less the subsidy payment up front to you
➤ no requirement for staff to take a fee each time the patient visits, thus saving time and making the appointment more pleasurable for everyone
➤ the legal contract is between the patient and the supplier providing the loan facility, so risk of non-payment to you is removed.

If you are planning to introduce this service to your patients, you will want to ensure it is being properly communicated throughout your practice. A practice with a patient co-ordinator is likely to have a greater take-up of extended credit facilities than one that does not. The co-ordinator has time to properly explain the advantages of the facility and to make all the necessary arrangements to apply for the loan. If you are relying upon associates to introduce the option of extended credit to the patient, you may find the number of patients actually taking up the option is reduced. This could happen for a number of reasons.
➤ The associate is not supportive of the scheme.

➤ The associate has not been fully briefed to discuss the scheme with patients.
➤ The practice team generally is not familiar with the benefits of the scheme.
➤ Information is not made readily available to patients by way of posters or information leaflets.
➤ The practice team has not been specifically instructed as to how and when they should introduce the facility to patients.

Monitoring the number of patients who do go ahead with extended credit facilities both as a practice average and per associate will provide you with an indication of how well the availability of the product is being communicated to patients. You should also be able to compare the take-up of treatment plans for the associates who do discuss this option with patients as opposed to those who do not. By illustrating the positive effect offering the facility has upon treatment plan take-up, you will be able to coach other associates to be predisposed to offer it to their patients.

Monthly direct debit plans

Offering a facility to patients to spread the cost of their routine care throughout the year can be a significant practice builder, particularly if your practice is converting or actively looking to develop a different profile of patients. It is imperative to introduce the means of monitoring the sign-up of patients onto these schemes to ensure the whole team is proactively informing and educating patients about the benefits of the plan.

If you are serious about developing a good source of predictable income (whether you are at the practice or not), you will want to track the number of new patient sign-ups; which members of your team are instrumental in those sign-ups, and whether the total numbers are in line with your target. You will also want to identify if any members of the team are not achieving the same level of sign-ups and address this with them in a one-to-one meeting. Failure to discuss the scheme with patients can be due to lack of confidence on the part of team members, lack of knowledge or lack of time. In the latter case, you may wish to assign a member of the team to be called upon to explain the scheme to patients. Otherwise, look at retraining those members of the team who are not meeting expectations.

The numbers of patients joining can be a good indication of their intention to stay registered at the practice for the foreseeable future – it's a vote of confidence in you and your team and as such a very important key performance indicator to the future health of your business.

If you have inherited a large capitation plan it is wise to audit the patients on the plan on a regular basis. It is one area of the business I make sure is covered when I carry out practice health checks.

There are several issues which may have a serious impact upon the profitability of your practice that are associated with capitation schemes. When a capitation scheme is introduced to a practice, it is often done as a mechanism to assist with a private conversion. If the conversion process has not been managed well, a proportion of patients can be placed in the wrong band, meaning they are paying insufficient fees to cover the cost of the dental treatment they are receiving. These patients often end up receiving treatment within this band for many years.

Another factor which can have a devastating effect upon profitability is the number of dental hygiene appointments that patients on capitation can have. The dentist refers the patient to the hygienist for a scale and polish. The hygienist notes some deep pockets and recalls the patient each quarter for further treatment, not realising that the patient is only entitled to two hygiene appointments per year in the band they are in. When this situation arises, the principal dentist not only provides hygiene services to the patient free of charge, he also pays his dental hygienist to provide them.

Case study

One practice I visited had only 84 patients registered on a capitation scheme. An audit carried out on 40 of these patients revealed that 26 were incorrectly banded and had collectively cost the practice £3,700 in treatment provided free. The dental hygienist was paid nearly £2,000 providing hygiene treatment for which no fee had been charged. When these figures were extrapolated upwards to estimate the total cost to the practice, the total figure reached almost £6,000. The principal dentist would have had to gross over £12,000 to cover this loss for every year that the problem was allowed to continue. Imagine the potential cost in a practice which has hundreds of patients on capitation!

There is also a risk of supervised neglect creeping in as a result of capitation and this risk needs managing and reducing by conducting clinical audits on a sample of patients within each band. Any principal dentist considering the purchase of a practice should conduct due diligence on any patient schemes to avoid the costs that may be incurred at a later date through supervised neglect.

Finally, check when the fees per band were last reviewed. It is easy to forget to raise fees annually to keep in line with increases in private fee per item.

Referral to specialists

This key performance indicator is very important and if your associate dentists rarely refer patients to specialists, you may want to carry out clinical audit programmes to ensure they are not overlooking the need to refer.

Some general practitioners operate at an exceptionally high clinical standard and often don't necessarily need to refer; however, as the practice owner, you will want to be sure this is the case and not that your associate is undertaking clinical work for which he or she does not have the necessary expertise and experience or that they are avoiding referral by not offering it as an option.

The patient should be provided with every possible option for treatment and in the case of a missing tooth this should include dental implants, even if the dentist treating the patient has to refer them on for this work.

If you have resident specialists, you will want to ensure sufficient internal referrals are generated from you and your associate dentists to ensure the specialist's time spent at the practice is productive and worthwhile. It also makes better commercial sense for the specialist to concentrate on the complex cases in order to release appointment time for the generalist. This is particularly relevant for endodontic treatment where a generalist can take much longer to carry out treatment – sometimes with a less predictable outcome.

New revenue streams can very successfully be developed through introducing specialist services into your practice. Specialist hourly rates are significantly higher than those of the generalist and patients are more likely to consider specialist treatment if they know they can receive it within the familiar surroundings of their own practice. The number of internal and external referrals going to the specialists provides an indication of the trend of the referrals part of your business and will help you to plan marketing and communications to patients and dentists to maximise the potential of this additional revenue stream.

To monitor the number of referrals, maintain a simple spreadsheet showing whom the referral came from, whom it went to, and what the outcome was.

Laboratory percentage to revenue

In financial terms, the expenses associated with laboratory work are classed as a cost of sale. The best way to judge whether your laboratory costs are in line with acceptable limits is to express the total cost as a percentage to revenue. The percentage will depend upon the profile of your practice, as a practice carrying out a great deal of implant work will record a higher percentage than a practice carrying out only a modest amount of restorative work.

It is not necessarily a positive indication if the lab work percentage is very low (say under 5%) of revenue as this often is a sign that there is very little restorative dentistry being carried out. At the other end of the scale, lab work showing as 15% of revenue is very high. A very low percentage could indicate that the lab used is of exceptional value; a very high percentage could indicate your practice is using an expensive laboratory because it provides superb results, but that these premium costs are not being passed on to the patient correctly.

To work out the percentage of lab costs to revenue, take the total amount of lab cost for a period of time, ensuring there are no outstanding bills and that there are no bills that relate to a different period. Then add up the total amount of revenue generated for the same period. Take the cost of the lab work and divide it by total revenue and then multiply by 100. This will give you laboratory cost expressed as a percentage of revenue. Carry out the same exercise for each associate working within the practice to check the practice average figure is not masking any issues relating to individual dentists.

As a practice, you should have a policy regarding the charging on of laboratory work to patients. Some practices use the lab cost as a basis for the cost of the whole treatment, applying a multiplying factor to the lab fee to arrive at the correct figure. Other practices charge an amount for the treatment and add the lab cost on top. It does not really matter how your policy works, as long as the cost of lab work is reflected in the fee. For example, if you have the policy that your associates can use any lab of their choice and one associate uses a lab which charges £100 for a bonded crown and another associates uses a lab which charges £150 for a bonded crown, you need to establish whether there is a justification – in terms of the quality of the work – to charge the patient a premium rate for the more expensive crown.

This needs careful consideration, not only to ensure that the needs of patients are consistently met but also because, from a commercial perspective, your business stands to have its profit margins eroded if you do not adjust the treatment fee in accordance with the lab fee.

It is also advisable not to take the overall percentage of lab costs to turnover at face value. What appears to be an average and acceptable ratio may be masking an issue that requires addressing.

Case study

I conducted a practice health check and found the lab percentage to gross revenue was 5.5%. However, I was concerned at the low hourly rate and low gross revenue of the practice and decided to take a sample of lab dockets and work out the percentage of each docket to the fee that had been charged to the patient. This revealed the total cost of lab work for these 10 dockets represented a huge 38% of the revenue generated. So although the total overall percentage seemed low, this was purely a reflection of the small amount of lab work being generated in relation to total turnover.

Example

Associate	Cost of lab work	Fee to patient	Lab percentage
Mr Smith	100.00	500.00	20.00
Mr Brown	135.00	500.00	27.00

This example shows that it only requires a slight increase of the lab fee to have a significant effect upon gross margin. If your turnover was £1 million, this example would reduce your gross profit by over £70,000.

Material costs percentage to revenue

The costs of dental materials to your business should be controlled by means of prudent stock control to ensure the levels of stock are adequate and the range of materials stocked allows for some flexibility and preferences for your associates. This may mean restricting the choices of composite material to two instead of having four or five.

Whilst it is good to shop around for best value, don't get drawn into letting a member of staff spend hours searching for bargains when a dealing with one preferred supplier will probably give you similar value and save a lot of time.

Some suppliers offer other incentives to use their services such as support for training, online ordering or price matching. Generally speaking, costs should be in the region of 4–6% of revenue providing this area of your business is being well controlled.

Staff salaries percentage to revenue

This is likely to be the single biggest overhead cost to your business and I generally come across huge discrepancies in this area, with costs running as low as 11% of revenue up to 28% of revenue. If you are concerned about your staff costs, there are a number of areas you can review to try to establish what the problem is.

It may be that your base staff costs are acceptable and it is your turnover that is low. This is often the case when a new practice opens and the business is building.

Some practices are understaffed and use agency staff on a regular basis to supplement their base staffing levels. This is a false economy and does not help to build a stable and committed team.

Again, practices that rely on more part-time staff may find they are over-compensating with staff hours and actually have an overlap of staff at certain times of the day.

On balance, I prefer to see a practice slightly overstaffed to allow for holidays and unforeseen circumstances to help keep stress levels in the practice down. Provided your team members are applying themselves to their work and there is no one coasting through their shift, this can give your business a long-term advantage in that it provides the necessary resource for your staff to spend time talking with patients about their treatment and care, and so drive revenue and good customer care standards.

CHAPTER 16

Interpreting and analysing the information

You or practice manager do not have to assimilate all the key performance indications of your business from the start. Use your profit-and-loss or management accounts as a starting point, looking first at revenue, then cost of sales, and finally overheads. Then use management reports from your patient management system or manual workings to gather other useful information.

Ideally, you need to be able to break down revenue per associate dentist or hygienist to enable you to analyse the overall contribution each is making to your business. Then you can start to draw occupancy percentage, hourly rates, conversion (treatment acceptance) and prescribing profiles into the picture to create an objective and detailed representation of where your business is productive and what areas require action to address performance issues.

Producing monthly management reports

Your practice manager should prepare all of this information in the form of a monthly report that you will both review together to discuss and decide what action is required the following month. All of the information provided within the report should help you establish whether the business is developing as desired and working towards achieving the objectives you set for your business at the start of the year.

The report layout is not important, provided it shows clearly and concisely the overall key performance indicators of the business and the breakdown per associate. Once you have completed your monthly management review meeting with your practice manager and have agreed on the areas that require action, your practice manager can proceed with arranging one-to-one meetings with the associate dentists to review their personal contribution to the business that month.

It is also useful to maintain a trend report that will show progress being made month by month to enable you to monitor growth. A trend report is also extremely useful in helping to predict future income and expenditure and can be used as a tool to help establish when recruitment for a new associate may be required, or refurbishment of a dormant surgery carried out to meet growing demand.

You or your practice manager should use the report to conduct one-to-one meetings with the associates and hygienists. This activity may seem a little daunting for your practice manager to begin with, depending on what level of authority she has over the clinicians and how much she is already involved in the financial performance of your business. If her role is more inclined towards managing the administration of the practice, it would be beneficial to review her skills and develop her knowledge of the business so she can play a key role in helping you to drive it forward. In the meantime, provide the support she will require to develop confidence in this extension of her role by accompanying her to the first few meetings. She will appreciate the support and your presence will reinforce the authority with which she is acting.

Associate dentists tend to react very positively to the opportunity to discuss their contribution to the practice on a regular basis. Often, poor performance is due to ignorance rather than lack of ability or poor attitude. The meetings also provide an ideal moment to integrate other areas of concern such as time keeping and their contribution to the team effort. The output from any report should always be presented using a positive and supportive style, with the key performance indicators being a factual basis used to commence a non-confrontational discussion. Facts are indisputable and therefore allow potentially sensitive topics to be covered without having to use a subjective or personal approach.

The specific key performance indicators of clinicians should only be shared with the clinician in question and any comparisons should be made only against practice averages. This will keep the information within a private arena where it cannot be used to name or shame any person's individual performance.

The primary objective from these one-to-one meetings is to share management information with associates and hygienists and agree which areas each one needs to focus on in order to perform to acceptable and agreed standards. The exercise may highlight further development needs, for example in communicating with patients for a dentist who has a low take-up of treatment plans by patients. It may reveal a concern relating to hourly rates which may be a symptom of poor prescribing profiles, poor interpersonal skills with patients or lack of confidence in completing restorative dentistry. Using the factual key performance indicators as a starting point facilitates discussions in potentially sensitive areas and allows all parties to consider the solutions in an objective and mutually supportive manner.

You may agree on several actions as a result of the meeting and review these areas again at the next planned meeting. With the right amount of application by the dentist and support from his or her team, you should be able to illustrate the improvement that has been made, which, in turn, encourages all parties to continue to work on those areas for continuous development. Should there be no improvement over an appropriate length of time, there may be a requirement to review the suitability of that associate or hygienist to your practice. Even if the most difficult decisions have to be made, you have the factual information and a record of meetings and suggested solutions to support you.

SECTION 6

Strategy, finance and planning – Keeping your eye on the end goal

'I think the most important CEO (Chief Executive Officer) task is defining the course that the business will take over the next five or so years. You have to have the ability to see what the business environment might be like a long way out, not just over the coming months. You need to be able to both set a broad direction, and also to take particular decisions along the way that make that broad direction unfold correctly.'

CHRIS CORRIGAN

Introduction

Business is constantly shifting and evolving, reacting to the needs and desires of consumers which, in turn, are influenced by changing trends, fashions and the advancement of technology and accessibility to the market place.

Consider the evolution that has taken place in people's shopping habits in the last ten years. The Dot Com revolution was heralded as a most significant development in IT communications with the development of the World Wide Web and Internet access, and it now represents a significant area of commerce where consumers choose to spend their time and money. This progression has fundamentally changed the way people buy and sell and allows unlimited access to information about products and services. Anyone who has access to the Internet can find out just about everything about anything and this huge medium has enabled consumers to educate and inform themselves without having to leave the comfort of their own home or office.

The outcome is a better-informed consumer market place, and consumers' aspirations are driven to higher levels, because they can see there are lifestyle choices to be made that will change their lives and which are within their reach.

The advent of the 'celebrity' has also had an impact upon the market. Consumers aspire to become the image of their favourite celebrity, dressing, behaving and even looking like their hero or heroine.

The fact that the desires and dreams of individuals often fall beyond their ability to pay for them is not a problem either. We now live in a world where it is acceptable to purchase everything you want and need on credit. The concept of not being able to purchase something until one has the money to buy it is defunct. Lending institutions start to target their market as soon as they can by offering students, whose earnings are limited, the opportunity to apply for credit. Consumers already in debt are offered the opportunity to increase their debt by taking out more loans or applying for new credit cards with alluring benefits.

How does business cope with these revolutionary changes in commerce and what effect does it have upon what we do to maintain and develop the business of dentistry so that we keep pace with the constant changes that face us?

As an ethical profession, dentistry cannot be seen to exploit the unrealistic aspirations of patients, and care must be taken to ensure treatments being offered are affordable and justifiable. However, just because treatment is not clinically necessary it does not mean it should not be carried out. As a dentist you are providing a service to your patients, and part of that service will include helping your patients to feel better about the way they look and the way they feel about themselves. As providers of a service the profession must react and respond to the changing needs of its patients and the business environment that the profession operates within.

This is why planning the future of your business is so important.

CHAPTER 17

Business planning

Where have you been, where are you now, where are you going?

From time to time it's good practice to remove yourself from the intensity of the day-to-day involvement in your business and stand back to review your progress and the direction you are heading in. Ask yourself some fundamental questions:

➤ Is my business heading in the right direction?
➤ Is my business evolving to meet the changing needs of my patients?
➤ Am I personally happy in my work?
➤ Am I managing my personal wealth and business finances to maximise return?
➤ On a scale of 1 to 5, what is my level of job satisfaction?
➤ Is my business progressive and dynamic or am I failing to make the changes necessary to move with the times?
➤ If I had the same opportunities, would I still be where I am today?

As we saw in Chapter 4, there is an intrinsic link between the aspirations we have in both our professional and personal lives. The roles we create for ourselves throughout our personal and working lives inevitably cross over into one another, and this means that key decisions about our future, whether they be the direction of our business or our work–life balance, have a knock-on effect in all our roles.

Assuming you have completed a 'health check' of your business following the advice set out in this book, and you have established its strengths and weaknesses, you will be in a much better position to start planning for the future. You will know which areas require improvement and development and what opportunities you are currently not making the most of. Your plan may be focused purely on developing the revenue or profitability of your existing business, or you may wish to change the profile of your business altogether by introducing new products and services, or even moving the location of your business.

The financial performance of a typical business plan that focuses purely on developing the potential of your existing business may look something like this:

Example: Anywhere Dental Practice business plan summary

Projected growth for the Anywhere Dental Practice in the next three consecutive years of 06/07, 07/08, 08/09:

06/07	£1.9m
07/08	£2.6m
08/09	£3.0m

Current key performance indicators

The practice is currently performing well against targets:

October	revenue £137.7k	Net profit £54.9k
November	revenue £153.9k	Net profit £42.9k
December	revenue £122.1k	Net profit £55.8k
January	revenue £156.3k	Net profit £49.1k

Current performance equates to 1.6m business over 12-month period

Current average hourly rate:

Hygiene	£74
Generalists	£145
Specialists	£261

Current average occupancy of providers:

Hygiene	72%
Generalists	72.5%
Specialists	70%

Current average utilisation of surgeries: 72%

Current actual spare capacity in days:
Anywhere Dental Practice is a 10-surgery practice. If we allow for 6-day trading, there are 60 days each week available. Currently surgeries are in use for 40.5 days per week, leaving 19.5 days spare for additional providers.

Current number of specialist referrals:

December	26
January	27

Current conversion rate (treatment plan take-up): 60%

New general patients:

December	6
January	16

Recalls:

December	82
January	220

TABLE 17.1 SWOT analysis

Strengths	Weaknesses
Clinical skills	Too reliant on key clinicians for revenue
Reputation	Lack of desire to grow business by key clinicians
Environment	Conversion percentage
	Administration
Opportunities	**Threats**
Marketing the practice	Increasing local competition
Implant business	Loss of general patients who don't like change
Introduction of new services	Loss of referring clinicians
HealOzone	
BriteSmile	
Referral base	
Self-referrals	
Clinical evenings	
Patient evenings	

2006/2007 Business development plan

Aim to grow the business by 19% based on 1.6m growing to 1.9m.
Equivalent gross revenue of 146k per month (not allowing for seasonal fluctuations).

WHAT
- Appoint Orthodontist initially 1 session every other week, building to 2 sessions per week. Target hourly rate £250 = 1k per session
  Commencing April
  Estimated contribution year 1: £35k
- Appoint Oral Surgeon initially 1 session every other week, building to 1 session every week. Target hourly rate £400 = £1600 per session
  Commencing April
  Estimated contribution year 1: £25k
- Increase conversion of referral patients to take up treatment to 70%
  Estimated increase in revenue: 50k
- Increase number of implant placements by 15% per month from July 2004
  January placements   26 = 65k
  February placements   33 = 82.5k
  March booked   30 = 75k
- Aim to place 35 to 40 implants per month from June – increased estimated revenue of 100k
- Increase Perio and Endo referrals by 15%

> Estimated increase in revenue:
  Perio   20k
  Endo   20k
> Encourage referrals to Periodontists for implants
  Estimated increase in revenue: 50k
> Increase General fees by 10% from 1 March, to £210 per hour
  Estimated increase in revenue: 25k
> Increase Hygiene occupancy to 80% and hourly rate to £80
  Estimated increase in revenue: 10k

HOW
> Implant explanation evenings held every six weeks
> Clinical study evenings held every six weeks
> Local display advertising on a regular basis budget required 12k
> Total marketing budget requirement 2% of turnover
> Development of local business network with similar client base
> Improve administration of referrals to drive conversion and dentist relation-
  ship
> Introduce 'friend get a friend' referral card
> Specialist newsletter to be distributed every quarter
> Newsletter mail shot to A, B and C1s in local and surrounding area

CAPITAL EXPENDITURE REQUIREMENT
Upgrade first-floor hygiene room to dental surgery: £1500
Install digital radiography: £3000
Replace chair in small hygiene room: £4000

2007/2008 Business development plan

Aim to grow the business by 28% increasing revenue from £1.9m to £2.6m.
Equivalent to 54k per week.

WHAT
> Continue to develop the Orthodontic and Oral Surgery referrals and self-
  referrals and increase sessions to 3 Orthodontic per week and 1 Oral Surgery
  per week
  Ortho @ £250 per hour @ 70% occupancy x 3 sessions per week (session being
  4 hours) = 80k
  Oral Surgery @ £350 per hour @ 70% occupancy x 1 session per week = 47k
> Specialists hourly rate £350 per hour @ 70% occupancy x 4 full-time equivalents
  = £1,764,000
> General dentists hourly rate £200 per hour @ 70% occupancy x 2 full-time
  equivalents = £504,000
> Hygiene hourly rate £85 @ 80% occupancy x 2 full-time equivalents = £240,000

HOW

➤ Similar marketing activity as in year 1 with greater emphasis on implants and referrals

➤ Total marketing budget requirement: 2% of revenue

➤ Target PCT for contracted-out Oral Surgery/Endo and Ortho

CAPITAL EXPENDITURE REQUIREMENT

➤ Create another implant suite either in existing perio surgery or in first-floor hygiene room

➤ Divide perio room to create additional hygiene room and upgrade ground-floor hygiene room to dental surgery

➤ Probable costs: 1 new chair and unit for new hygiene room – 8k

➤ Upgrade ground-floor chair: 2k

➤ Building works to divide perio room, move cabinetry, chair and unit and make good – to be confirmed

2008/2009 Business development plan

Aim to grow the business by 15% from £2.6m to £3m.
Equivalent to 62.5k per week.

WHAT

➤ Continue to develop the Orthodontic and Oral Surgery referrals and self-referrals and increase sessions to 4 Ortho per week and 2 Oral Surgery per week
Ortho @ £250 per hour @ 70% occupancy x 4 sessions per week (session being 4 hours) = 134k
Oral Surgery @ £350 per hour @ 70% occupancy x 2 sessions per week = 94k

➤ Specialists hourly rate £350 per hour @ 70% occupancy x 4.5 full-time equivalents = £1,984,000

➤ General dentists hourly rate £200 per hour @ 70% occupancy x 2.5 full-time equivalents = £630,000

➤ Hygiene hourly rate £80 @ 70% occupancy x 2.5 full-time equivalents = £252,000

HOW

Similar marketing activity to that of previous years, with a 2% marketing budget.

A more radical plan may incorporate more fundamental changes and could include bringing on board a partner, moving premises, buying an additional business or selling the business altogether.

Before beginning to draw up your tactical plan, make sure you have considered whether these key aspects of your business have also been reviewed. In other words, can you still achieve the desired outcome of your business plan over a five-year period if you are still the sole owner of the business, or will your plans require some additional investment that may require you to consider offering a partnership to an associate?

If there are other considerations such as the question of incorporation or perhaps taking on an expense-sharing partner, now is the right time to include these factors in your long-term plan.

Many practice owners I know find it challenging to stand back and plan for the future, and it could be beneficial to bring in a third party who can advise you independently about the choices you have to make now that may make a difference to your future, both in a professional and personal sense. These may take the form of a specialist accountant, independent financial adviser or solicitor. There are various associations of specialists to dentists, including the National Association of Specialists to Dentists and the Association of Specialist Practitioners to Dentists. Professional organisations have to meet strict criteria to become members and all have specialist knowledge and interests in dental businesses in their specialist field.

CHAPTER 18

Dental business structures

Introduction

In this chapter, Alan Suggett, BSc (Hons) FCA, from Baker Tilly Tax and Advisory Services LLP provides an interesting insight into the different ways of structuring dental businesses and the relative tax implications. Alan Suggett is a member of the National Association of Specialist Dental Accountants (NASDA) and he has successfully been advising dentists and dental business owners for many years.

There are currently three ways in which a dental business can be operated. These are: as a sole trader, a partnership or a 'corporate body'. Until July 2006 the last option was not permitted (with the exception of a small number of corporate bodies which were allowed several years ago).

Sole traders and partnerships

Traditionally dental businesses have therefore been operated as either a sole trader or a partnership. Both of these methods share many characteristics, the two most critical being firstly the basis of taxation of profits (both sole traders and partnerships are dealt with under the income tax self-assessment rules), and secondly, unlimited liability for the dental business owners. In the case of partnerships the liability situation is even more severe as the concept of 'joint and several liability' applies. In other words, each partner can be bound by the actions of another partner. In simple – but slightly unrealistic – terms, this means that a partner could take delivery of a Rolls Royce in the partnership name under credit terms, and then disappear to South America leading to the remaining partners being liable to repay the finance company!

In more recent times, a hybrid of sole trader and partnership has frequently been used – this is an 'expense-sharing arrangement' or an 'expense-sharing partnership'. It is fair to say that there is considerable confusion, even within the professional adviser community, regarding the technical status of these two methods of operating a dental business. In a properly constituted 'expense-sharing arrangement', the dental business owners are not in partnership; they are a collection of sole traders who share certain expenses (e.g. property costs). In the case of an 'expense-sharing partnership', the entity is legally a partnership, but the profit shares of the individual partners are calculated by means of a formula which usually varies directly with their own personal working contribution. There are also expense-sharing arrangements which technically are partnerships as the expense sharers share, for example, profits generated by associates working within the practice. A definition of a partnership is 'persons carrying on a business in common with a view to profit' and therefore by this definition the 'expense sharers' can, in fact, be partners. However, what difference does this make in practice? The answer is, other than in extreme circumstances, none at all!

Sole traders, partnerships and expenses sharers all benefit from flexibility, a minimal amount of 'red tape', and a favourable capital gains tax position on the sale of the business (as they are normally able to take advantage of business asset taper relief which can bring the effective rate of tax on gains down to 10%). The disadvantage of these structures is taxation of profits at the income tax highest rate once the basic rate band has been used up; an inability to bring non-dentists into business ownership (e.g. spouses) as this is illegal, and practical difficulties in selling small portions of the business to others (e.g. associates). Some commentators would also highlight unlimited personal liability as being a significant disadvantage of this method of business ownership. In some dental businesses this could be an important factor. However, the operation of a dental business – unlike that of most other types of business – usually brings negligible personal risk. The worst that could happen to a typical dental practice is that unusual circumstances would cause it to cease trading in an organised manner, without the extreme losses which sometimes occur in other commercial situations.

It is fair to say that dental practices have been operating on a self-employed basis in one of the above structures for many years without any problems. Dentists, like any other business owners, complain about paying a lot of income tax but, in reality, the current UK top rate of tax (40%) is relatively modest compared with rates that have applied in the past.

Corporate bodies

In July 2006 the law was changed in two important ways. Firstly, dental businesses were allowed to be operated through 'corporate bodies'. Secondly, where a corporate body is used, the majority of 'directors' must be registered Dentists or Dental Care Professionals.

There are a number of interesting consequences of the above two changes; let's look at them.

➤ Business owners. There is no reference at all to business owners, only directors. It is perhaps worthwhile explaining that in the case of a limited company (where the people who control the affairs of the company on a day-to-day basis are called *directors*) directors are not necessarily the same people as shareholders. The conclusion therefore is that *anyone* can be a shareholder in a dental corporate body operated by a limited company. In other words, external investors can own a dental corporate body as long as the majority of the people who control it on a day-to-day basis (i.e. the directors) are Dentists or Dental Care Professionals.

➤ Other types of corporate body? The law allows operation of a dental business through a corporate body, but no definition of a corporate body is given. The obvious one, as mentioned above, is a limited company (which is controlled by directors). However, other professions (e.g. lawyers and accountants) make wide use of Limited Liability Partnerships (LLPs). LLPs are controlled by 'members' – they do not have directors. Is it therefore correct to say that LLPs are not allowed to operate dental businesses? There is no clear answer to this, but the consensus amongst professional advisers is that LLPs are permitted and the wording in the legislation is not intended to exclude them – it is just sloppy!

Finally, there is another type of corporate body which in commerce generally is extremely rare. It is an 'unlimited company'. Unlimited companies share all of the characteristics of a limited company, apart from the fact that the shareholders have unlimited liability with regard to the company's affairs. In return for the shareholders taking on this potentially onerous condition they are allowed to keep secret all of the company's financial information. Why on earth would a dentist wish to consider this option? Perhaps the option might be considered by an NHS dentist who wishes to exploit the tax advantages of incorporation, but does not want his extremely large profits to be obvious to the outside world!

So what type of dental business is likely to find the prospect of incorporation attractive, and what type of corporate body should be used?

We are still at a relatively early stage in our experience, but it is fair to say that there are very few situations where LLPs are thought to be useful. When comparing LLPs with a partnership, the tax position is broadly similar, but an LLP brings with it the advantage of limited liability for the business owners. As indicated above, this is not usually likely to be an important factor.

Unlimited companies have a certain but limited attraction, as previously highlighted.

By far the greatest use is likely to be made of limited companies.

So far the most frequent use of a limited company has been made in an attempt to reduce the overall taxation charge on profits. Corporate tax rates are lower than the higher rate of income tax (for tax year 2007/08, the small-company rate of corporation tax (on profits up to £300,000) is 20% and will rise over the next two years to 22%). Further details of other taxation aspects are shown below.

Other than tax savings, it is likely that limited companies will benefit those dentists who wish to involve associates (or even staff generally) in partial business ownership. Historically, involving an associate in business ownership has usually been an 'all or nothing' event. One day an associate, the next day a partner. In future, by a gradual transfer of limited company shares, it will be possible for associates to have, initially, a small proportion of company shares, building this up over a number of years. There are tax-effective arrangements which can make this route even more attractive.

Limited companies also permit external investors to inject funds into the dental business for expansion purposes. This could be on an informal basis where friends of the dental business owners invest, or alternatively, more formally, investment by specialist investors, such as venture capital funds, injecting significant amounts to enable a dental business to expand rapidly. There are two particularly tax-effective ways to structure third-party investment: the Enterprise Investment Scheme for individuals, and Venture Capital Trust funding, which is a form of institutional investment. Venture capital funding is not likely to be exploited by many dentists, but it could be a route to a huge growth in business value for those who have the desire, appropriate vision and entrepreneurial flair to take successful advantage of it.

Turning back to the more typical reason for incorporation, what are the issues which need to be considered?

Whilst there isn't a standard formula for evaluating whether or not incorporation will save tax on profits, it is fair to say that, if all of the profits are extracted, incorporation will not usually be advantageous for very profitable multi-partner practices. This is perhaps surprising, but financial feasibility studies indicate that this is the case. It may be that the position will change in future, particularly if the 'mainstream' corporation tax rate is reduced further. For some years the mainstream corporation tax rate has been set at 30%, but this was reduced in the March 2007 budget to 28% from 1 April 2008. There is a school of thought that believes this is part of a downward trend to, say, 25%, at which point the incorporation of very large practices may well be beneficial.

There are also problems at the lower end of the scale for NHS practices. The way in which an NHS dentist's pension is calculated within a corporate body is different from the calculation of the pension of a sole trader or partnership. It is not possible to go into detail in this analysis, but this will mean that incorporation of an NHS practice is almost certainly not worthwhile unless profits per principal are comfortably in excess of the 'earnings cap' for superannuation purposes (currently approximately £110,000).

For those practices with profits between the two extremes outlined above there is some potential for tax savings by incorporation. This arises in the following way:
➤ lower tax rates on retained profits
➤ sale of goodwill to the limited company
➤ repayment of loans more tax effectively
➤ involvement of spouses (perhaps!).

Once again it isn't appropriate to go into great detail about this as it is very important to be guided through the process by an experienced professional adviser. However, the basis behind these savings is as follows.
➤ Goodwill. When goodwill is sold to the limited company, the gain, in most circumstances, is taxed at 10% taking advantage of 'business asset taper relief' for capital gains tax purposes. A loan account is created within the new limited

company which is drawn off over a number of years in substitution of income which would otherwise be taxed at the highest rate of income tax. It is, however, worthwhile to point out the potential difficulty which can arise in valuing goodwill for tax purposes, and the special attention which HM Revenue and Customs are currently giving to this area.

➤ Repayment of loans. In an unincorporated dental practice the capital element of loan repayments comes out of income which has been taxed at the highest rate of income tax. When a limited company repays a loan it is out of income which has been taxed at a lower rate. In this way, a substantial tax saving is achieved.

➤ Involvement of spouses. Under appropriate circumstances, it can be beneficial from a taxation point of view for the spouses of the dental business owners to become shareholders in the limited company. If the company then adopts a strategy of distributing some of the profits by way of dividends to shareholders, and the spouses have unused basic rate tax allowances, then the overall level of income tax paid can be reduced. However, this area is rather a moving target as HM Revenue and Customs do not like taxpayers saving tax by splitting income with their wives.

If at this stage you are thinking, 'This all sounds rather complicated, is it really worthwhile?' The answer is, 'Possibly!' However, it is certainly fair to say that six-figure savings can be made as a consequence of incorporation, but you must tread very carefully.

Of course there is more to consider in life than taxes, and therefore many other factors need to be taken into consideration when deciding whether incorporation is appropriate for a dental practice.

Even if the circumstances of the dental business are appropriate now, who is to say what will happen in the future? It will be pointless benefiting from a tax saving now only to see it unravelled and have even more tax to be paid if a corporate structure is disadvantageous at some time in the future.

At the time of writing this commentary, the attitude of Primary Care Trusts (PCTs) to incorporation is still uncertain. Whilst it is inevitable that PCTs will allow dental corporate bodies to contract with them, the terms of the contracts are uncertain. In particular, will PCTs insert a 'change of ownership' clause when contracting with a corporate body? In the absence of such a clause it will be possible for the shareholders of a limited company to sell their shares to someone else and, because the contract is in the name of the company and the company itself hasn't changed, the benefit of the contract will pass to the new shareholders. In this way the contract will have been 'sold' to another party without the involvement of the PCT. Contrast this with the case of a non-corporate body, where the PCT must approve the transfer of a contract from one dentist to another when he sells his business. This feature of corporate bodies is seen to be attractive to dentists in that it is a way for them to preserve their goodwill. The simple insertion by the PCT of an appropriate clause into corporate body contracts would prevent this from happening.

Then there is the question of sale of the dental business. Currently when a non-corporate-body dental business is sold, it is simply the sale of assets from one dentist to another (e.g. goodwill, fixtures and fittings, and perhaps a property). In order to preserve the initial tax advantages gained by use of a limited company it will be necessary for the selling dental business owner to sell the shares in the limited company to the purchaser. Whilst this arrangement is quite common in non-dental businesses (and earns attractive due diligence fees for corporate finance accountants!) it is unheard of for dental businesses which have been incorporated since the law changed in 2006, as at least two years should be allowed from incorporation to sale to take advantage of Business Asset Taper Relief for capital gains tax purposes. It is unlikely in the long term that this will cause problems on the sale of dental businesses, but it is an added hurdle in the sale process.

In this section a flavour has been given of possible different ways of owning and operating a dental business, and also some of the advantages and disadvantages. Unfortunately it is impossible to give a thorough guide in an overview of this type and, as indicated previously, it is absolutely vital for dental business owners to receive legal, accounting and taxation advice about the type of structure which is most appropriate for their circumstances.

Alan Suggett BSc (Hons) FCA
Baker Tilly Tax and Advisory Services LLP
1 St James' Gate
Newcastle upon Tyne
NE1 4AD
www.bakertilly.co.uk

CHAPTER 19

Personal and professional wealth management

Introduction

In this chapter, Simon Fitton from Baxter Fensham provides information and advice on the importance of managing business and personal finances together in order to maximise the benefit of lifelong financial planning. Simon Fitton from Baxter Fensham is an expert in wealth management and the practice has advised dental practice owners for many years, helping them to maximise the value of their professional and personal investments. Here Simon provides sound advice showing why practice owners should be considering the management of their personal and professional finances together and what they should be taking into consideration, together with what the desired output should be.

Business and personal financial planning

This book highlights the importance of management information and reporting, making possible a more efficient and profitable business model. The result of getting this right makes for a more enjoyable working environment for all the staff, as we all feel in control. It means that we can set time aside to work both 'in' and 'on' our businesses, and to look at the kind of lifestyle that we would wish to enjoy, now and in the future, away from our places of work.

One of the major pitfalls of financial planning is that business owners continually separate business from personal, but the reality is that they are inextricably linked. There are valuable tax reliefs available through a business, that are different from the personal tax regime, but so often these are captured at the expense of the others. Furthermore, by seemingly providing a solution within a business, a problem may be compounded when one's personal finances are considered. Let's consider some of the issues.

➤ How many business owners rely on the sale value of their businesses to provide a retirement income when they stop work? Does goodwill exist today? Do you

own the property that you operate from?
➤ How can an owner extricate monies from the business now, and what are the tax implications?
➤ Should I incorporate? What are the financial benefits of this action?
➤ What impact will the new contracts have on my earning ability, and what are the implications of my practice moving away from the NHS to a fully private practice?
➤ How many businesses have restrictive partnership agreements in place? Do they even have a partnership agreement, and if so, how would it cater for one partner's family in the event of him or her having a long-term illness or even dying?

In 2006, there was a change to pension regulations called 'simplification' and this brought with it greater clarity and flexibility, together with much larger contribution scope. However, there was also a lifetime limit introduced, and if your pension fund exceeds this limit, then there will be penalties to pay!

Some of these issues are not new, but they have a renewed layer of importance attached by dint of regulation changes. It is so important that you talk with specialists that understand the nuances peculiar to your profession, and to that end, personal and business planning should be aligned.

What kind of lifestyle can I have?

Yes, this must always be your starting point, as you need to quantify what it is you want from your life so you can prioritise how to achieve your objectives. Remember that a want is distinctive from a need. One may NEED food, clothing and shelter but may WANT caviar, luxury goods and a holiday villa. We are not all the same and, indeed, not everyone is materially aspirational; some may prefer a more conservative protection of accumulated wealth.

Some questions you could start asking yourself could include:
➤ What you do away from work? Any plans to take up other hobbies or interests in the future? What is stopping you doing them now?
➤ How do you feel about your job? Is it a necessary evil or do you really enjoy what you do? How do you see the future as far as work is concerned?
➤ What does retirement mean to you? For example, if you are in good health, will you keep working even though you could afford to retire?
➤ Will your retirement be a well-earned extended holiday?

After interrogating yourself about what you want from your life, it is vital that you create a 'context' for any planning that you do. One of the most powerful and empowering tools available to you through an independent financial planner is a 'Cash-flow Modelling Analysis' or 'Lifeplan'.

Create a Lifeplan

You need to understand the relationship between what your objectives are, the amount of risk you are comfortable with and how much money you are prepared to commit. These are the strategic decisions that you need to consider.

The first thing to do is to organise your current affairs into a financial plan. You should be given tools to help you determine what you will be spending your monies on at different stages of your life. This demonstrates how far your existing arrangements go towards helping you achieve your financial goals. It will also enable a planner to identify areas of weakness and vulnerability. The most important purpose that this exercise serves is that it helps identify and quantify any shortfalls you may have in your planning as it stands.

The next stage is to meet to reaffirm your objectives by interrogating your cash-flow model. This would outline the strategy you should adopt to achieve your objectives. This will incorporate wealth creation, using a structural investment process, or wealth preservation to ensure that, once financial independence is achieved, your position is protected.

This plan would then need to be underpinned with insurances to guard against illness or death; you don't want your plans to fail because of this.

Investment solutions and wealth management

Mark Twain once said 'There are two moments in a man's life when he should not speculate: the first is when he does not have the means, the second is when he does.'

You need a financial planner to help you to manage the relationship between the risk of your portfolio and the amount of money you need to invest to achieve your objectives. It therefore goes without saying that the more successful your investment experience is, the happier you will be with your planning in general. This can be achieved by:

➤ varying the ratio of equities to short-term bonds to meet your risk tolerance
➤ spreading risk as far as possible through Global Diversification
➤ using a mix of Domestic, Foreign and Emerging Market funds
➤ using short-term, lower-risk, high-quality bonds to meet known or probable cash needs.

You could construct a huge roulette wheel of the hundreds of active fund managers out there and 'gamble' on which one will have predicted the **right** firms, in the **right** sectors, in the **right** markets, at the **right** time and will do it consistently EVERY year. Alternatively, you could simply take advantage of the vast amounts of academic research that has won Nobel Prizes, costs less and is bespoke to your individual requirements.

Risk plays an integral part in financial planning. A dictionary definition of risk is:

'the possibility of suffering harm or loss; danger'.

When most people think of risk associated with money they think of the negative. This is probably because we are conditioned to think of risk in terms of loss. After all, if someone says something is risky, they don't tend to see the positive side! However, there is a positive side to risk. Every day on the stock market money managers are using tools to reduce the amount of risk involved.

➤ No risk, no reward. There is no such thing as a risk-free investment. In order to build assets, you must undertake some type of risk. Greater potential return is the reward for undertaking greater risk.

➤ Choose appropriate risks. Know and understand the risks involved in various savings and investment vehicles. Make sure you are comfortable with the risk level of the investments you choose.

➤ Manage risk, do not try to avoid it. Diversify: holding a variety of investments and shares lessens the negative impact of an investment that performs poorly. Invest over time to offset market fluctuations. Monitor your investments to be sure that the risk/reward guidelines you have set have not changed.

➤ Maintain a long-term perspective. Plan to own funds over a long time to help lessen the effects of price fluctuations and market volatility.

The problem with defining risk is that your personal definition will be based on your experiences, knowledge and perception of what risk is and what it means to you. Only when you sit back and think about what level of risk you are comfortable with will you be able to reach a happy medium.

The less risk you take the more likely you are to achieve your objectives, but you'll need to invest more money to get there. Conversely, if you take a higher level of risk you are less likely to achieve your objectives, but you'll need to invest a lower amount to reach your goals.

In summary, reaching your goals and objectives is driven by getting the balance between the level of risk you are willing to take and the amount of money you have available to invest.

Why a financial planner may help

No one can guarantee you investment success, but a well-thought-out, sensible investment plan tailored to your unique needs can greatly improve your probability of meeting your future financial goals.

Appointing the right financial planner will give you the freedom and peace of mind to pursue more rewarding activities with loved ones. The planner will:

➤ help you create an overall investment strategy that reduces costs, minimises risk and maximises returns

➤ serve as a partner and guide to help you make important financial decisions

➤ work with your accountant, lawyer and other professionals to protect your assets and interests

➤ deliver easy-to-read and easy-to-understand investment and performance reports

➤ provide you with ongoing investment education
➤ establish open communication and access to personal and objective advice
➤ help you to become financially well organised
➤ consolidate your financial arrangements to simplify your life.

How to pay your planner

Commission-based advisers such as banks, insurance companies, investment managers, stockbrokers and the vast majority of financial advisers are not equipped to assist people with investing. The commission-based pay structure of the industry sets up a conflict of interest. It could be argued that the traditional model of commission-based compensation invites adviser abuse, with their clients as their victims.

What good is advice, if it's not objective? Unlike stockbrokers who have every incentive to maximise commissions and costs, a fee-based financial planner will have strong incentives to minimise your costs and maximise your account value.

The result is that you have a service that is more proactive, more holistic in terms of the areas covered and more comprehensive in terms of the level of advice that is being given. It will only work, however, if you have complete trust and faith in the impartiality of the advice and service being given. It will not work if the adviser has to sell you something to get paid nor will it work if what you buy determines the amount the adviser earns.

A commission-based service places both the client and the adviser in the vulnerable position where one of them will nearly always be compromised. The only way to ensure the impartiality of the advice and the service is to make it fee based.

Hopefully, this brief overview has given you an insight into the importance of planning your finances with your two 'hats' on. Your business activities can be driven by a specific plan to inform your personal life, which must surely come first. It is then a matter of how you use your business to make it possible to meet your personal aspirations.

Ensure that your advisers have the ability, facilities and commitment to your care to apply this degree of analysis. If done correctly, you should not find yourself out of your depth. Neither should you find yourself walking away from opportunities that would be reasonable for you to seize.

The above information should be considered for guidance only, to improve awareness; and it is **not** intended as, nor should it be taken as, specific advice. The points mentioned are only summaries of what are complex areas; therefore, before taking any action, you should seek advice from a professional adviser.

The author, Simon Fitton, is a director and fee-based financial planner with Baxter Fensham Ltd, which is authorised and regulated by the Financial Services Authority. sfitton@ baxterfensham.com (www.baxterfensham.com).

CHAPTER 20

Conclusion

Introduction

All of this activity not only allows you to focus the direction of your team to ensure your business is growing at the pace you ideally want it to, it also means you are fully prepared when it comes to planning your exit strategy and the quality of life you want to realise when you retire.

The goodwill value of your business is based on revenue and profitability and you will ensure you receive the financial rewards you deserve if you have planned for and managed your exit strategy well.

Many businesses fail to realise their full potential due to poor planning and execution of those plans. Although there may seem to be plenty of time before you sell your share of the business, you never quite know what the future holds in store and it's preferable to be in a position to sell at a premium when you want to – or perhaps have to – rather than accept a smaller return on your lifetime's work because you haven't planned to maximise your return.

Ensure practice health check keeps on working for you

Once you have completed your first practice health check, or brought in someone to do it for you, you will find change really does become possible. The actions that result from the audit can generally be completed within a 12-month period. The most important thing is to maintain a focus on achieving the changes and developments to improve your business over that period. And once you have completed the changes you have identified, you should be re-grouping and redefining your objectives for the next 12-month period, so that the process becomes a continuous cycle of improvement and development. This means you and your team should be regenerating the focus and impetus each year by taking a day out to develop your business plan for the next 12 months.

The health check in itself will add no value to your business. It is what you do with the results that count. Of all the clients for whom I have completed practice health checks, only one has reported that the exercise was not valuable.

Upon investigation to establish the reason why, it became apparent that none of the recommendations made in my report had been acted upon and the practice owner had not acknowledged that the issues were a direct result of their poor management of their business.

Perhaps the most important factor to bear in mind before you embark on a health check is that you may find the most major change that has to take place in your business lies within yourself. The change may be needed in the way you approach the running of your business; how you interact with patients and your colleagues; how you organise your time to ensure you are an effective and focused leader, and knowing when to accept help from experts who will work with you to help you succeed. Be prepared to accept that some of what is going wrong in your current situation probably comes down to you and however unpalatable that realisation may be, change will only be possible if you acknowledge that fact.

We all underestimate the effect that we have upon the individuals who fall within our circle of influence. As managers of others it's easy to offload the responsibility if a task is not completed properly or if a patient is unhappy about the service they have received. If something is wrong in your business, always be prepared to reflect upon your involvement in the situation first and to consider whether you have failed to provide the right direction or instruction. If you do not take responsibility for your role in ensuring your business works well, how can you expect your team to do the same? In the first part of the book we focused a great deal on the management of the team and how a well-trained and focused group of people can make a huge difference to the success of your organisation. Leaders of good teams are good leaders – luck does not come into it.

The aim of the health check is not to identify all the things that are going wrong and then find someone to blame. The whole process is designed to reflect objectively across the whole spectrum of what makes your business tick and establish opportunities to improve and develop those areas. You can then put into place a plan to follow up your findings with actions to ensure the output is a more productive, profitable and cohesive team that delivers superior products and services to your patients.

I hope this book has provided you with an insight into how you can make a difference in your practice and how the proactive management of your team could add untold value to your business and improve the quality of your working life.

Benchmark your Practice

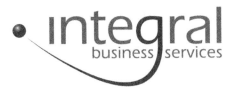

> Have you sat down recently and really thought about how your business functions?
> Which areas are generating the most profit for you?
> Where are your costs too high?
> Why can't your team do what you want them to do?
> Which of your associates is adding the most value?
> How can you double your revenue?
> How can you market your practice without spending a fortune?
> Why are there so many issues every day?
> Where are the hidden costs that affect your profitability?
> Want to know the answer to these questions?
> Spend five minutes completing the attached Benchmark exercise.
> Then talk to us about our comprehensive Business Health Check Service.
> The Benchmark Audit is divided into the key areas of your business.
> The audit is designed in a quick-tick format so you can complete it in around five minutes.
> It will provide you with an indication of the 'health' of your business.
> It could be the most valuable five minutes you invest in for your business.

HOW TO COMPLETE THE BENCHMARK AUDIT

Tick the appropriate boxes and be completely honest with yourself.

Tick column No. 1 if you answer 'no' to the question, if you don't know or if you are not satisfied with your current situation.

Tick column No. 2 if you can answer 'yes' to the question but are not sure you are using the information/process to its full potential or if you believe it could be improved.

Tick column No. 3 if you can answer 'yes' to the question and are confident you could not improve it in any way.

* Tick this column if you feel this area is a particular issue in your practice

TABLE 20.1 Practice health check

Benchmark Audit	*	1	2	3
Key area 1. People:		✓	✓	✓
Your people are your most important asset				
PRACTICE MANAGER				
Do you have monthly business review meetings with your practice manager?				
Does your practice manager present key performance indicators to you?				
Does your practice manager execute your marketing plan?				
Does your practice manager understand your vision for the practice?				
Does your practice manager take full responsibility for the operation of the practice?				
Would you describe your practice manager as a business manager?				
STAFF				
Are you satisfied with the recruitment process of your auxiliary and reception team?				
Are you satisfied with the current levels of staff retention?				
Do you have a staff appraisal system in active operation?				
Do you have a formal structure for performance management?				
Do you have a formal absence and attendance policy?				
Do your staff have job descriptions, key responsibilities and personal objectives?				
Do your staff understand your vision for the practice?				
Do your staff have contracts of employment?				
ASSOCIATES				
Do you know what proportion of treatment is private for each associate?				
Do you know how many patients are referred to the hygienist?				
Do you know what the prescribing profile is of your associates?				
Do your associates understand your vision for the practice?				
Do your associates contribute to the team spirit in your practice?				
Do you know that your associates are maintaining cross-infection control standards?				
Is the clinical standard of care offered by your associates to your requirements?				
Are your associates up to date with CPD?				
Do you know what gross and net productivity each associate is contributing?				

cont.

Benchmark Audit	*	1	2	3
Key Area 2. Customers:		✓	✓	✓
Your customers and the experience you give them are the future success of your business				
Have you devised a 'patient journey' to ensure excellent consistent customer service?				
Do you carry out regular customer service surveys?				
Do you monitor and constantly review your product and service offering?				
Do you have a complaint recovery procedure?				
Do you spend time talking with your customers?				
Do you spend time listening to your customers?				
Do you have a method to record comments made by customers?				
Does the team receive training in customer service skills?				
Do you have a policy statement on customer service standards?				
Key Area 3. Systems/ Procedures/Operations:		✓	✓	✓
Processes underpin your business				
How many recalls are sent a month? How do you know?				
Is your current level of debt acceptable? What percentage is it to turnover?				
Is your current level of 'fail to attends' acceptable? What percentage is it to turnover?				
Is your current level of late cancellations acceptable? What percentage is it to turnover?				
Have you got a system to manage lab work effectively in and out of the practice?				
Do you know you are receiving best value from suppliers?				
Do you have a daily maintenance procedure for chairs and units and hand pieces?				
Key Area 4. Management information:		✓	✓	✓
Key performance indicators				
Do you know the average hourly rate of your practice?				
Do you know the hourly rate of each clinician including hygienists?				
Do you know the occupancy percentage average of your practice?				
Do you know the occupancy percentage of each clinician?				
Do you know how many patients opt for private treatment?				
Do you know the average value of private treatment?				
Do you know the percentage of material costs to revenue?				
Do you know the percentage of lab costs to revenue?				
Do you know the percentage of staff costs to revenue?				

cont.

Benchmark Audit	*	1	2	3
Do you know your gross and net profit percentage?				
Do you know how much profit you make from tooth whitening?				
Key Area 5. Marketing:		✓	✓	✓
Maximise the opportunity to promote your business				
Do you know how many new patients have registered in the last three months?				
Do you know how they came to hear about your practice?				
Do you know what return on investment your marketing activity has delivered?				
Do you advertise in Yellow Pages?				
Have you a functioning, up-to-date website?				
Have you a practice brochure?				
Do you send a welcome pack to every private patient?				
Do you use the local press for PR opportunities?				
Do you maximise the opportunity to promote to customers inside the practice?				
Do you offer interest-free payment facilities?				
Do you offer an accident and emergency product?				
Are patients on your capitation practice plan under constant monitoring and review to ensure they are in correct band and only receiving treatment permitted within their band?				
Do you carry out regular audits on your direct debit plans?				
Key Area 6. Finance/Strategy/Planning:		✓	✓	✓
Keeping your eye on the end goal				
Do you regularly use the services of an Independent Financial Adviser to manage your business and personal finances?				
Do you have a strategic two-, three- and five-year plan?				
Do you have an exit strategy?				
Do you develop and implement an annual business plan?				
Do all your associates have personal development plans for the next 24 months?				
Key Area 7. Quality Assurance System:		✓	✓	✓
Measure, monitor and improve for sustained growth and profitability				
Do you have a system to ensure all statutory and legal requirements are adhered to?				
Do you have a health and safety policy?				
Do you have a policy for cross-infection control?				

cont.

Benchmark Audit	*	1	2	3
Do you have a policy for manual handling?				
Are you completely happy with your ionising radiation policy and procedures?				
Do you have documented policies and procedures?				
Does the practice partake in operational and clinical audits?				
Does the practice have a peer-review meeting?				
Do you hold regular team meetings?				

If you have marked more than one tick in column No. 1 and No. 2 in any key area, your practice could benefit from a Business Health Check. www.integralbusinessservices.co.uk

Index

Printed and bound by CPI Group (UK) Ltd, Croydon, CR0 4YY

23/10/2024

01777681-0001